Healthy-Aging Diet

What You Eat Can Help You Live Healthier and Longer

2020 Report

A Special Report published
by the editors of *Tufts Health & Nutrition Letter*
in cooperation with
The Friedman School of Nutrition Science and Policy
Tufts University

Cover image: © franckreporter | Getty Images

Healthy-Aging Diet: What You Eat Can Help You Live Healthier and Longer

Consulting Editor: Diane L. McKay, PhD, Director of Tufts University's Friedman Online Graduate Certificate Programs,
Assistant Professor in the Friedman School of Nutrition Science and Policy and the Tufts School of Medicine

Author: David Fryxell
Creative Director, Belvoir Media Group: Judi Crouse
Editor, Belvoir Media Group: Dawn Bialy
Production: Mary Francis McGavic

Publisher, Belvoir Media Group: Timothy H. Cole
Executive Editor, Book Division, Belvoir Media Group: Lynn Russo Whylly

ISBN 978-1-879620-69-8

To order additional copies of this report or for customer-service questions, please call 877-300-0253, or write: Health Special Reports,
535 Connecticut Avenue, Norwalk, CT 06854-1713.

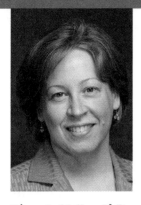

Diane L. McKay, PhD

Director of Tufts University's Friedman Online Graduate Certificate Programs, Assistant Professor in the Friedman School of Nutrition Science and Policy and the Tufts School of Medicine

There has never been a more important time to adopt science-supported dietary strategies to protect your health as you age. Daily, we see headlines about America's obesity epidemic, the rise in type 2 diabetes, the prevalence of cardiovascular disease and cancer, and the looming threat of an explosion in cases of Alzheimer's and other forms of dementia. While no dietary pattern can completely protect against these conditions associated with aging, choosing to eat right—along with physical activity—can improve your odds.

The current *Dietary Guidelines for Americans* (DGA) are unequivocal in the message that even small changes in what you eat and drink can benefit your health. Shifting to healthier eating patterns can help bring about lasting improvements in health, according to the *DGA*.

Change Your Pattern, Change Your Life. The guidelines emphasize the importance of overall healthy dietary patterns, rather than focusing just on individual foods or nutrients. Such patterns include a Mediterranean-style diet, the DASH eating plan, and a vegetarian regimen. We'll explore some of these options in this book, which focuses on ways to adjust your diet to achieve a healthier eating pattern.

This book also emphasizes a healthy eating pattern that meets the unique needs of older adults. These are reflected in the MyPlate for Older Adults, developed at Tufts University and its Jean Mayer USDA Human Nutrition Research Center on Aging. This eating pattern forms the underpinning of this book, although we also discuss other healthy patterns.

Science for Smarter Choices. Even the MyPlate for Older Adults, which is customized to the nutritional needs of seniors, is not a "one-size-fits-all" plan, however. The aim of such a plan—and of this book—is to provide informed options for healthier eating. Throughout these chapters, we give science-based examples of smart choices that can be part of a healthy dietary pattern. But if you love tuna and loathe salmon, or enjoy spinach but can't stand kale, that's okay. Go ahead and customize the advice in this book to your tastes and budget.

We will also remind you about some of the less-optimal foods to avoid or limit. Our focus, however, is largely on the positive: tasty, nutritious food choices that can enrich your diet and your life. We'll explore the fantastic variety of vegetables and fruits and introduce you to whole grains you might not have tried. Other chapters will look at smart selections in the dairy case and weighing the pros and cons of foods high in protein; we've also added a chapter on protein sources you might be overlooking, such as seafood and plant foods. If you bought into the "all fat is bad" fad, you'll be glad to learn that not all fats affect your body in the same way, and some fats actually have beneficial health properties. You might also be surprised to learn that some beverages have benefits similar to certain plant foods.

Keeping Up. We also recognize that the advice in this book may change in the future. That's the essential nature of science—and all of these recommendations, like the *DGA*, are based on the latest nutritional science. What we know is ever evolving as scientific research continues to pull back the curtain on our understanding of our bodies and the world around us. This evolution is reflected in the "New Findings" boxes scattered throughout these pages, which offer updates on the latest research.

The frontiers of what we know about diet and healthy aging are continually expanding. This book will help you keep up and learn how eating right can improve your odds of living healthier longer. I look forward to accompanying you on this exciting journey to healthy aging.

Diane L. McKay, PhD

TABLE OF CONTENTS

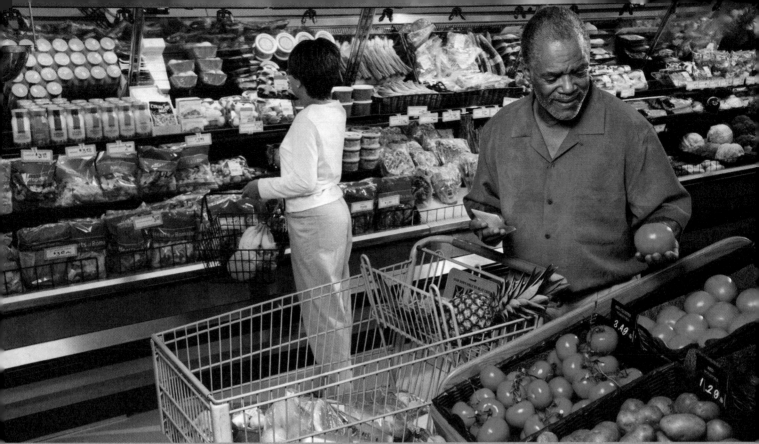

© Iofoto | Dreamstime

New Findings

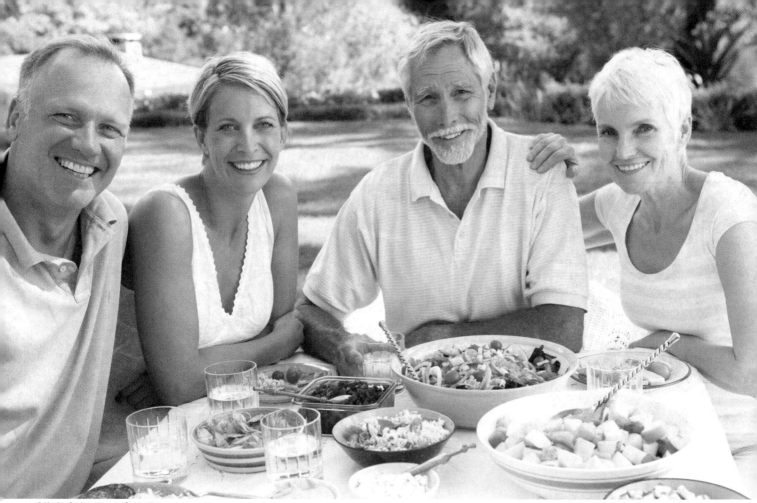

Following a healthy diet can help you reduce your risk of chronic disease and manage conditions you may already have, such as high blood pressure and high LDL cholesterol.

NEW FINDING

Eat Better, Live Longer

One of the largest surveys of data on global dietary habits and longevity adds powerful evidence to the link between eating well and living longer. Consuming more vegetables, fruit, fish, and whole grains was strongly associated with longevity. The researchers also reported that approximately one-fifth of deaths worldwide were associated with poor diets that were high in added sugars, salt, and trans fat, and contained fewer vegetables, seeds, and nuts. The findings suggest that, if people who consumed poor diets had instead been following healthy diets, an estimated 11 million deaths could have been avoided in 2017. Of the 195 countries analyzed, the U.S. ranked 43rd in diet-related deaths. France, Spain, and Peru were among the countries with the fewest diet-related deaths, while Papua New Guinea, Afghanistan, and the Marshall Islands ranked the worst. The authors concluded that encouraging the addition of healthy foods to the diet rather than advising people to reduce consumption of unhealthy foods is a better strategy for reducing mortality.

The Lancet, April 3, 2019

1 The Nutrition You Need Now

As you get older, you may find yourself agreeing with the words of baseball legend Satchel Paige: "If I knew I was going to live this long, I would have taken better care of myself." Experts estimate that half of all American adults—almost 120 million people—suffer from preventable chronic diseases, primarily conditions associated with aging.

The good news about getting older is that it's never too late to start taking better care of yourself. The first step is to increase your level of physical activity. The latest physical activity guidelines, updated in December 2018, call for most adults to get at least 150 minutes of physical activity weekly, incorporating some strength-building exercise along with aerobic activity.

The second step to healthy aging is to make wise dietary choices. It's clear that what you eat and drink can strongly affect your health, both negatively and positively. The benefits of choosing the right components in your diet are often overlooked, since it's easy to get caught up in all the "don'ts" and the damage that can be done by an unhealthy diet. Eating right also can be a particular challenge for older adults, since you need fewer calories as you get older. That means it's important to choose foods that are nutrient dense—packed with vitamins, minerals, fiber, and other essential nutrients. And you may need to boost your intake of certain nutrients, because your body's ability to absorb nutrients decreases with age.

Tufts experts have created a MyPlate for Older Adults graphic (see page 10) that focuses on these special nutritional needs. The elements of this graphic form the organizational basis of this book, which will show you how to take these simple nutritional strategies and make them part of your everyday life.

Eat Right for Life

Shifting to healthier food choices can decrease your risk for chronic diseases such as cancer, type 2 diabetes, and heart disease—all of which are more common in older than younger adults. Eating healthier also can help you manage a variety of health conditions, including high blood pressure, high LDL cholesterol, elevated blood glucose, and digestive disorders. A healthy dietary pattern paired with an active lifestyle can even help protect against the more subtle but no less devastating loss of lean muscle mass associated with aging, a condition for which Tufts scientists coined the term "sarcopenia" in the late 1980s. Once thought to be an inevitable accompaniment to advancing years, sarcopenia is now understood to be largely preventable.

Research by Renata Micha, PhD, RD, an assistant professor at Tufts' Friedman School, and colleagues recently reported that eating more of certain foods and not enough of others was associated with nearly half of all deaths in the U.S. due to cardiometabolic diseases and events that include heart disease,

Obesity Linked to Increased Cancer Risk

Looking for more motivation to maintain a healthy weight? A new report from the World Cancer Research Fund (WCRF) links obesity to 12 types of cancer. The report analyzed a decade of research to develop cancer-prevention recommendations. It found strong evidence that being overweight or obese throughout adulthood increases risk of cancer of the mouth, esophagus, stomach, pancreas, gallbladder, liver, colon, breast (post menopause), ovaries, endometrium, prostate, and kidney. The prevalence of obesity is increasing worldwide, the report noted. To reduce cancer risk, the WCRF recommends being physically active, eating a diet rich in whole grains, vegetables, fruit, and beans; and limiting consumption of fast foods, red and processed meats, sugar, and alcohol. The report also advises getting nutrients from foods rather than supplements.

Diet, Nutrition, Physical Activity and Cancer: A Global Perspective, 2018

stroke, and diabetes. That amounts to about 320,000 deaths a year, or nearly 1,000 deaths each day.

"To reduce the risk of premature death from cardiometabolic disease, our data suggest Americans need to eat more fruits, vegetables, nuts, seeds, whole grains, vegetable oils, and omega-3-rich fish," Dr. Micha says. "At the same time, people need to cut back on salt, processed meats, and sugar-sweetened drinks."

Not surprisingly, this advice echoes the dietary recommendations of Tufts' MyPlate for Older Adults, as well as many of the principles underlying other healthy eating plans we'll look at, such as the Mediterranean-style and DASH diets.

Key Ingredients

Dr. Micha's research showed that certain dietary factors were associated with deaths from certain diseases. For example, deaths caused by heart disease was most strongly associated with low intake of nuts/seeds and seafood, and high intake of processed meats, sugar-sweetened beverages, and sodium. The most deaths from stroke were associated with low fruit and vegetable intake and high sodium intake. The most deaths from type 2 diabetes were associated with low intake of whole grains and high intake of processed meats and sugar-sweetened beverages.

10 Dietary Factors and Mortality

According to a study published in the *Journal of the American Medical Association* in 2017, 10 dietary factors contribute to more than 45 percent of cardiometabolic disease (CMD) deaths. Ranked individually, these factors are:

DIETARY FACTORS ASSOCIATED WITH INCREASED MORTALITY	% OF ANNUAL CMD DEATHS
High in sodium	9.5
Low in nuts/seeds	8.5
High in processed meat	8.2
Low in seafood omega-3 fat	7.8
Low in vegetables	7.6
Low in fruits	7.5
High in sugar-sweetened drinks	7.4
Low in whole grains	5.9
Low in polyunsaturated fat	2.3
High in unprocessed red meat	0.4

The analysis also showed that the number of deaths declined among people who consumed more nuts/seeds and polyunsaturated fats and fewer sugary drinks, while the number increased for those who consumed more sodium and unprocessed red meats.

Diet vs. Disease

If you need more evidence to back up the link between your health and your diet, consider a report from the Centers for Disease Control and Prevention that said five of the 10 leading causes of death for individuals over age 60 are conditions that benefit from diet and nutrition intervention. Besides raising your risk of dying, all five of these conditions—cardiovascular disease, cerebrovascular disease, type 2 diabetes, cancer, and kidney disease—also affect your quality of life and your ability to live independently.

Cardiovascular Disease

Three risk factors for cardiovascular disease—the leading cause of death in the U.S. and around the world—are influenced by diet: unhealthy blood lipid levels (including high LDL cholesterol and triglycerides), high blood pressure (hypertension), and obesity. Cardiovascular diseases include coronary artery disease, heart disease, peripheral arterial disease, heart failure, and atrial fibrillation, among others. These diseases can cause heart attacks, pulmonary embolisms (blood clots in the lungs), and deep vein thrombosis (blood clots in the legs).

Cerebrovascular Diseases

These are conditions that develop as a result of problems with the arteries that supply blood to the brain. The most common types of cerebrovascular events are ischemic and hemorrhagic strokes. Inadequate blood flow to the brain also can also cause vascular dementia. The most important risk factor for cerebrovascular diseases is high blood pressure, which can be affected by dietary sodium intake as well as obesity.

Type 2 Diabetes

Characterized by high blood glucose (sugar) levels in the bloodstream, type 2 diabetes is associated with a two to four times higher risk of death from heart disease or stroke. Other complications from diabetes include vision loss, kidney disease, and neuropathy (nerve damage, usually in the legs and feet). Maintaining a normal weight and controlling

Physical Activity Guidelines for Americans

The second edition of the *Physical Activity Guidelines for Americans*, which was released in late 2018, continues to call for at least 150 minutes of moderate-intensity aerobic activity, like brisk walking or fast dancing, each week. Adults also need muscle-strengthening activity, like lifting weights or doing push-ups, at least two days each week. The guidelines also added some new emphases for adults:

- Move more and sit less. New evidence shows a strong relationship between increased sedentary behavior and increased risk of heart disease, high blood pressure, and all-cause mortality.

- Evidence also shows that physical activity has immediate health benefits, including reducing anxiety and blood pressure and improving quality of sleep and insulin sensitivity.

- Long-term physical activity helps prevent eight types of cancer (bladder, breast, colon, endometrium, esophagus, kidney, stomach, and lung); reduces the risk of dementia (including Alzheimer's disease), all-cause mortality, heart disease, stroke, high blood pressure, type 2 diabetes, and depression; and improves bone health, physical function, and quality of life. For older adults, physical activity also lowers the risk of falls and injuries from falls. For all ages, physical activity reduces the risk of excessive weight gain and helps maintain a healthy weight.

- Other evidence shows that physical activity can help manage health conditions that Americans already have. Exercise can decrease osteoarthritis pain, reduce disease progression for hypertension and type 2 diabetes, reduce symptoms of anxiety and depression, and improve cognition for those with dementia, multiple sclerosis, ADHD, and Parkinson's disease.

your intake of foods and beverages high in sugars and carbohydrates can help you manage your blood glucose levels. And eating more fruits, vegetables, and whole grains is recommended to help control the complications of diabetes, as well as prevent or delay its onset.

Cancer

Research suggests that eating whole and minimally processed foods contributes to a reduced risk of cancer. Experts advise limiting red meat and processed meat and eating more fruits, vegetables, and whole grains to reduce your risk. It's also important to maintain a healthy weight, since obesity has been linked to a higher risk of several types of cancer. According to the American Cancer Society, as many as one-third of all cancer deaths in the U.S. are related to diet and activity factors.

Chronic Kidney Disease

With chronic kidney disease (CKD), your kidneys cannot properly filter waste and excess fluids from your blood. When waste products and excess fluids remain in your body, they can cause swelling and high blood pressure, impair the function of your cardiovascular and immune systems, and/or increase your risk of bone fractures. The chances of developing CKD increase with age; it most commonly affects individuals age 70 and over. People who have diabetes, hypertension, cardiovascular disease, and/or are obese—all conditions related to diet—have a higher risk of CKD. On the other hand, a healthy diet and keeping yourself hydrated can reduce your risk.

Be Smart About Nutrients

Making healthy choices at every meal can help you get the nutrition you need to reduce your risks of chronic disease. That starts with breakfast, according to researchers who found that people who ate their biggest meal at breakfast were more likely to be leaner, as measured by Body Mass Index (BMI), than those who ate the most at lunch or dinner. Breakfast eaters also tended to maintain a healthier weight than those who skipped breakfast.

These breakfast findings align with recent advice from the American Heart Association, which noted that skipping breakfast is linked to greater risks of obesity, impaired glucose (blood sugar) metabolism, and diabetes.

Know Your Nutrient Density

Those recommendations don't mean you should simply add calories to your breakfasts without subtracting elsewhere. In fact, as we've noted, as you get older, your overall need for calories declines if you are less physically active, as is typical for the majority of older adults. You might also eat less because of a poor appetite, illness, or medication side effects. With fewer calories going in, it's especially important to get the most nutritional "bang" for your caloric "buck." That's why nutrient density is so important.

What's the difference between nutrient-dense foods and nutrient-poor foods? A large peach and five ounces of non-diet cola both contain about 65 calories, but the peach contains fiber, vitamins A and C, potassium, and other nutrients—it's more nutrient dense. The cola is energy dense, or high in calories, because of its added sugar content—about 15 grams of sugar, the equivalent of almost four teaspoons—but it provides no healthy nutrients. In addition, eating a peach will help curb your hunger, but the cola will not; your body doesn't register beverages as fuel in the same way it does solid foods.

Nutrient-dense foods include fruits, vegetables, whole grains, beans, nuts, seafood, lean poultry and meat, dairy products, and eggs. Most popular snack foods, such as potato chips, corn chips, and cookies and crackers made from refined grains are less nutrient-dense. In general, nutrient-dense choices are more likely to be whole foods rather than highly processed foods.

Even within the fruit and vegetable categories, some foods are more nutrient-dense than others; for example, substituting fresh spinach for iceberg lettuce can boost your nutrient intake. The same is true when choosing grains: Brown rice, for example, has almost six times more fiber and more magnesium, selenium, and manganese than the same amount of white rice, and whole-wheat flour is higher in fiber and several B vitamins than unenriched white flour.

A Fresh Start for Your Plate

Nutrient-dense food choices are essential to MyPlate for Older Adults. The icon depicts a colorful plate with images to encourage older Americans to follow a healthy eating pattern along with physical activity. The plate is composed of:

- 50 percent fruits and vegetables
- 25 percent grains, most of which are whole grains
- 25 percent protein-rich foods, such as fish, poultry, lean meat, beans, nuts, and fat-free and low-fat milk, cheese, and yogurt.

The icon also shows good sources of fluids, such as water, milk, tea, soup, and coffee, and heart-healthy fats, such as vegetable oils and vegetable oil-based spreads. Tufts experts also advise using herbs and spices in place of salt to lower your sodium intake.

Little by Little

Diets that require drastic changes are usually unsuccessful in the long run,

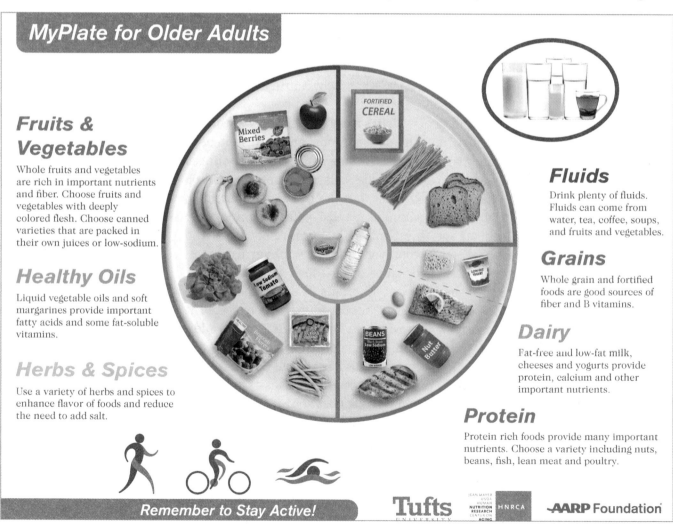

MyPlate for Older Adults

Fruits & Vegetables

Whole fruits and vegetables are rich in important nutrients and fiber. Choose fruits and vegetables with deeply colored flesh. Choose canned varieties that are packed in their own juices or low-sodium.

Healthy Oils

Liquid vegetable oils and soft margarines provide important fatty acids and some fat-soluble vitamins.

Herbs & Spices

Use a variety of herbs and spices to enhance flavor of foods and reduce the need to add salt.

FORTIFIED CEREAL

Mixed Berries

Low Sodium Tomato

BEANS

Nut Butter

Fluids

Drink plenty of fluids. Fluids can come from water, tea, coffee, soups, and fruits and vegetables.

Grains

Whole grain and fortified foods are good sources of fiber and B vitamins.

Dairy

Fat-free and low-fat milk, cheeses and yogurts provide protein, calcium and other important nutrients.

Protein

Protein rich foods provide many important nutrients. Choose a variety including nuts, beans, fish, lean meat and poultry.

Remember to Stay Active!

Tufts UNIVERSITY

JEAN MAYER USDA HUMAN NUTRITION RESEARCH CENTER ON AGING HNRCA

AARP Foundation

which is why Tufts experts advise you to start by making small shifts in your food and beverage choices. For example, switch to whole-grain pasta and choose whole-grain bread instead of white bread for sandwiches. Snack on fresh fruit rather than cookies. Eat fish for dinner once a week for starters, or go meatless on Mondays.

Making these small changes and sticking with them is the best approach to long-term improvements in eating habits. Once your initial healthy changes become habits, make a few more changes. If you plan on making major changes in your diet, talk with your primary health-care provider first.

The power of this long-term approach has been proven by research showing that improving diet quality over at least a dozen years is associated with lower total and cardiovascular mortality. People who eat more whole grains, vegetables, fruits, nuts, and fish, and less red and processed meats and sugary beverages, may significantly reduce their risk of premature death.

When selecting foods, keep these strategies in mind:

▶ **Make it easy to make healthier choices.** Put a bowl of apples on the counter and keep cut-up fruits and ready-to-eat veggies handy in the fridge. Portion out plastic bags of celery, baby carrots, grapes, and grape tomatoes at the beginning of the week so they are ready to grab and go.

▶ **Canned and frozen fruits and vegetables store well and are convenient**—just avoid those that contain added salt and sugar. If varieties packed in sugary syrup or salty fluids are the only products available, give them a quick rinse before serving.

▶ **Choose reduced-sodium varieties of soups,** broths, and condiments.

▶ **Replace sugar-sweetened beverages** with homemade flavored water by adding slices of lemon, lime, orange, or cucumber or sprigs of mint to a pitcher of water.

▶ **Replace highly processed snacks** like chips and pretzels with air-popped popcorn or unsalted almonds and walnuts.

▶ **Try a small portion of dark chocolate** to satisfy your sweets craving and skip the cookies, cakes, candy, and desserts that are high in added sugar.

▶ **Make a list before going to the grocery store and stick to it.** You might want to avoid entire aisles in the supermarket—generally, the perimeter of the store is where you'll find the least processed, most nutritious foods.

▶ **When you're eating out,** do some research first: Many chain and fast-food restaurants provide complete nutrition information on their websites. When you're at a restaurant that doesn't provide nutrition information, ask your server how dishes are prepared and what ingredients they contain. Many restaurants allow some customization of entrées; for example, ask for pasta with olive oil and garlic rather than alfredo sauce.

MyPlate for Older Adults also promotes regular physical activity with icons depicting common activities that include daily errands and household chores. Although some of those chores do not take the place of more formalized exercise routines involving cardiovascular activities, the chores are included to remind older adults that there are many options for regular physical activity in everyday life.

Nutrients of Note

Another important reason to choose nutrient-dense foods is because, as you age, you're more likely to be lacking certain key nutrients. We'll look at some reasons for nutrient shortages in a minute, but first, let's look at the nutrients that are of particular importance for older adults.

Calcium

Calcium is vital to maintaining bone density and preventing fractures. This mineral is needed in increased amounts by women over age 50 and for all adults over age 70. Because there are some possible side effects from high levels of calcium in supplement form, experts advise getting as much of your daily calcium needs as possible from dietary sources.

Vitamin B$_{12}$

The amount of B$_{12}$ your body needs for proper blood cell formation, neurological function, DNA synthesis, and other tasks doesn't change with age, but your body's ability to extract this vitamin from food might decrease. That's because older adults often produce less stomach acid or take medications that decrease acid production. Vitamin B$_{12}$ is bound to proteins in foods such as meat, fish, poultry, eggs, and dairy products, and stomach acids normally help release the B$_{12}$ for your body to use.

The synthetic form of vitamin B$_{12}$ found in fortified foods such as breakfast cereals or used in supplements is already in a form that doesn't require stomach acid for your body to use it. If a blood test reveals that you are deficient in B$_{12}$, your doctor will likely recommend B$_{12}$ supplements.

Vitamin D

Vitamin D is essential for bone health, since it aids in the absorption of calcium and it blocks a hormone that causes bones to become brittle. Vitamin D also plays a role in immune function, brain health, insulin regulation, muscle strength, and many other vital processes. Your skin naturally makes vitamin D when it is exposed to sunlight, but this ability declines with age and older people often spend less time in the sun. People who live in northern climes can't make enough vitamin D in the winter because there's not enough ultraviolet light.

You also get vitamin D from certain foods, but it can be difficult to obtain in adequate amounts from dietary sources alone. Only a handful of foods naturally contain vitamin D, including some types of fish, whole eggs, and some mushrooms. Some foods and beverages, including many brands of milk, orange juice, and breakfast cereals, are fortified with vitamin D.

Fiber

When you get older, the organs and systems in your body, including the

---

Non-Dairy Sources of Calcium

Even if you don't or can't consume dairy products, you can get the calcium you need. Choose alternative "milk" products fortified with calcium, and include some of these foods in your meal plans:

- **Breakfast foods.** Fortified whole-grain cereals deliver 100 milligrams (mg) or more calcium per cup.

- **Nuts and seeds.** Some nuts are relatively high in calcium, notably almonds (96 mg per quarter-cup), hazelnuts (39 mg), pistachios (32 mg), and walnuts (30 mg). Some seeds also provide calcium; poppy seeds have 126 mg per tablespoon, chia seeds, 90 mg per tablespoon, and sesame seeds, 88 mg per tablespoon.

- **Fresh fruit.** One medium orange (one cup) contains 52 mg of calcium. (A cup of fortified orange juice has about 300 mg of calcium, but choose whole fruit more often than juice and avoid juice drinks with added sugars.) Kiwifruits have even more calcium, with 61 mg per cup.

- **Dried fruit.** Figs (120 mg per one-half cup) and dates (58 mg per one-half cup) can help you hit your calcium goals.

- **Beans and lentils.** Top choices include white beans (80 mg per one-half cup), navy beans (63 mg), kidney beans (58 mg), pinto beans (52 mg), and edamame (49 mg).

- **Leafy greens.** One cup of cooked spinach contains 245 mg of calcium, and one cup of cooked collard greens contains 268 mg. Kale has about 177 mg of calcium per cup cooked, bok choy has 158 mg per cup cooked, and mustard greens have 165 mg per cup cooked.

- **Other veggies.** One cup of cooked, mashed sweet potato contains 77 mg of calcium. Other orange-fleshed veggies also deliver calcium with 90 mg in a cup of acorn squash and 84 mg in butternut squash. One cup of cooked broccoli has 60 mg, while its cousin, broccoli rabe, has 100 mg per cup cooked.

- **Seafood.** Canned fish get calcium from edible bones: There are 325 mg in 3 ounces of sardines and 212 mg in 3 ounces of salmon. Some other seafood varieties also can contribute calcium, with 78 mg in clams and oysters, 77 mg in shrimp, 73 mg in wild rainbow trout, and 50 mg in king crab. (All numbers are for 3 ounces of cooked seafood.)

- **Tofu.** Calcium amounts in tofu vary by brand and by the substance that's used to firm it up—anywhere from 150 to 430 mg per one-half cup. Tofu prepared with calcium sulfate has the highest calcium content, and some tofu is fortified with calcium; check the Nutrition Facts label and the ingredients list.

gastrointestinal tract, function less efficiently. This means constipation is more likely—but getting enough dietary fiber can help. Adequate fiber intake also has been linked to lower risks of several diseases associated with aging, including cardiovascular disease, diabetes, and colorectal cancer. When you increase your fiber intake, do the same with your fluid intake; water helps keep waste moving through your intestines.

Zinc

Tufts research has suggested that getting adequate zinc may help strengthen older adults' immune systems. Zinc supplementation has been associated with an increase in the function and numbers of T-cells—white blood cells that target and destroy invading pathogens, such as bacteria.

The Effects of Medications

Older people tend to take more medications—between three and five prescription drugs each, on average—plus over-the-counter drugs. Medications can interfere with your body's ability to utilize nutrients by decreasing the absorption, availability, or storage of nutrients, as well as by increasing the amount of nutrients that are excreted. These are some of the most common medications that affect the nutrients you need:

‣ **Anti-hypertensives.** Medications for high blood pressure called diuretics can decrease the availability and increase the elimination of zinc, as well as increase the excretion of B vitamins, potassium, magnesium, and calcium; examples include Diuril, Microzide, and Lozol.

‣ **Bronchodilators.** Medications delivered via an inhaler for asthma and other respiratory difficulties increase the excretion of calcium and block vitamin D absorption; examples include Symbicort, Dulera, Serevent, Ventolin, and Proair.

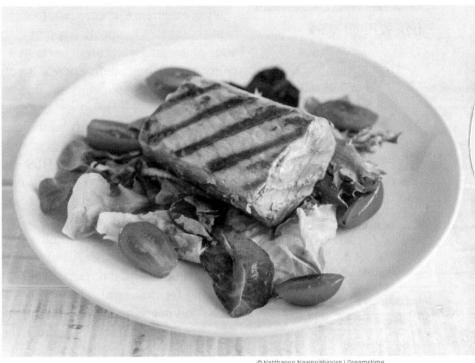

© Natthapon Ngamnithiporn | Dreamstime

Fatty fish, such as tuna (above) and salmon, are good sources of vitamin D.

‣ **Proton-pump inhibitors (PPIs).** Drugs used to treat heartburn and gastroesophageal reflux disease by decreasing the production of stomach acid can negatively affect the absorption of vitamin B_{12}, vitamin C, calcium, magnesium, iron, and zinc; examples include Aciphex, Nexium, Prevacid, and Prilosec.

Other Reasons for Shortages

The health conditions for which you might be taking medications also can affect your nutrient intake. These include heartburn or reflux, depression, a thyroid disorder, and nausea or loss of appetite from chemotherapy or other medical treatments. As you age, you might also experience changes in your sense of taste or smell, poor dentition, and difficulty swallowing—all of which can affect nutrition.

Dietary adjustments often can address some of these factors. Another possibility is that some elderly adults have more difficulty shopping for and preparing healthy foods due to reduced mobility, vision loss, and lack of transportation.

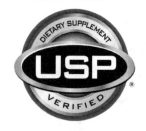

USP Verified Mark

How can you be sure a supplement contains what the label promises? One way is to look for this seal, which indicates that the supplement has been tested by the U.S. Pharmacopeia and found to contain the ingredients on the label in the declared strengths and amounts. Supplements that are USP verified also have been found to be free of potentially harmful contaminants, and have been created in sanitary conditions and by well-controlled processes in accordance with FDA and USP Good Manufacturing Practices.

If you experience unintentional weight loss and/or loss of appetite, report it to your physician, who can order tests to check for nutrient deficiencies. If you need to increase your nutrient intake, you may want to consult a registered dietitian to help you modify your diet.

Cautions on Supplements

At any age, consuming a healthy diet is the best way to get the nutrients you need. It may be tempting to pop a pill to boost your intake of vitamins and minerals, or as "insurance" against deficiency, but most research reports disappointing results from nutrients in pill form. This suggests that it's difficult to replicate the benefits obtained from the nutrient mix present in whole foods.

About 40 percent of American adults take multivitamin and mineral supplements. Studies have shown that users of such supplements have higher blood levels of vitamins A, C, D, and E and several B vitamins. However, research has not proven that taking a multivitamin decreases your risk of heart disease, cancer, or other health conditions.

Calcium and vitamin D supplements are taken by many older people in an effort to keep their bones strong. However, one review that included an analysis of data from 33 previous trials totaling more than 51,000 people ages 50 and older concluded that people who took calcium supplements, with or without extra vitamin D, were no less likely to suffer fractures than those who didn't use supplements.

Similarly negative findings may cause you to rethink fish oil supplements that promise to deliver heart-healthy omega-3 fatty acids. One combined analysis of 10 large randomized trials reported that fish oil supplements were not associated with significantly reduced risks of heart disease, heart attacks, or other major coronary or vascular events.

An exception to the thumbs-down on supplements is vitamin B_{12}, as noted above. If you're deficient, your body can more readily absorb the synthetic form of B_{12} found in supplements and fortified foods.

If you've considered boosting your nutrient intake with drinks or "shakes," you're also probably better off bypassing them. The American Geriatrics Society (AGS) has advised against using the popular liquid supplements, even for older adults who are suffering from unintentional weight loss.

Supplement Safety

One key to safe use of supplements is taking only the amount that will correct your deficiency; most people do not need mega-doses. If your doctor recommends supplementation, get clear instructions on what type and dosage of supplement you need.

Check with your doctor before beginning any supplement regimen. It's also critical to inform your doctor about any supplements or other over-the-counter products you are already taking, as supplements can interact with many medications. For example, if you take warfarin (Coumadin) to prevent blood clots, taking high doses of vitamin K or fish oil supplements may increase your risk of bleeding.

When choosing any type of supplement, exercise caution: Testing has revealed that some supplements contain more or less of the active ingredient(s) listed on the label and/or potentially harmful substances. Look for the "USP Verified Mark" on the label—this means the supplement has been tested by the U.S. Pharmacopeia.

Instead of relying on supplements, you can protect your health as you age in a safer and far more delicious way. The dietary patterns we'll explore in the next chapter and the healthy foods we'll highlight throughout this book are flavorful as well as nutritious.

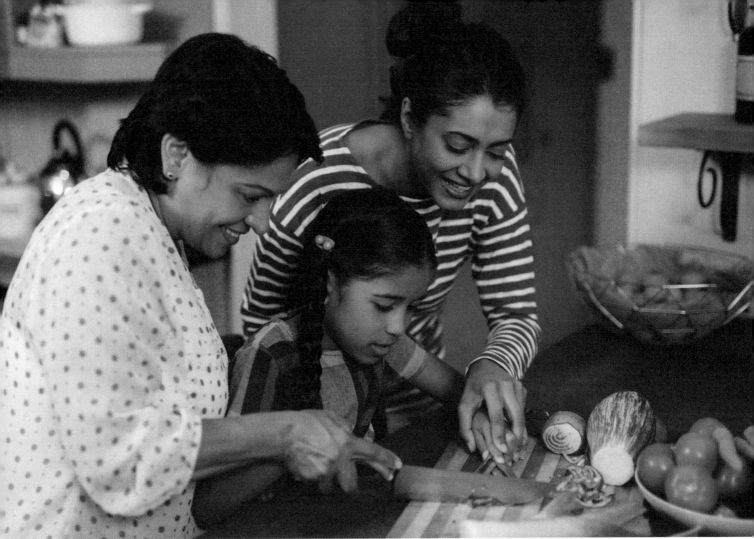

2 Dietary Patterns for Life

The 2015-2020 *Dietary Guidelines for Americans* (DGA) is now being updated to align the recommendations with the latest nutrition science. But it's a good bet that, whatever else changes, the emphasis on healthy eating patterns introduced in the current DGA will remain. The key to nutritious eating, according to that expert guidance, is following an overall healthy dietary pattern rather than focusing on individual foods or nutrients.

A Healthy Eating Pattern

Your entire diet, including what you eat and drink and how much you eat and drink, is important for achieving and maintaining a healthy body weight, obtaining adequate nutrients, and reducing the risk of chronic disease. A healthy eating pattern isn't achieved just by eating more of one or two foods and less of a few others. According to the DGA, a healthy eating pattern includes:

- A variety of vegetables, including dark-green, orange, and red varieties
- Fruits, especially whole fruits
- Grains, at least half of which are whole grains
- Fat-free or low-fat dairy, including milk, yogurt, cheese, and/or fortified soy beverages
- High-quality protein foods, including seafood, poultry, legumes (beans, lentils, and peas), eggs, lean meat, nuts, seeds, and soy products
- Oils, including olive, canola, corn, peanut, soybean, and sunflower oils

Cooking and eating at home makes it easier to follow a healthy eating pattern and helps you avoid dietary downfalls found in highly processed foods, such as added sugar, high sodium, and empty calories.

A healthy eating pattern also limits saturated fats and trans fats, added sugars, and sodium. Let's look more closely at what this means for your dietary choices.

Healthy Fats, Not Fear of Fats

If you still think of all fats as bad for you and always choose low-fat products—even if they are otherwise high in sugar or refined carbohydrates—you're behind the times. In recent years, the low-fat fad has been discredited and the scientific consensus regarding dietary fat has changed. Nutrition experts now emphasize that different fats affect health differently, and the total amount of fat you consume is not as important as the types of fat you consume. Reflecting this change in expert opinion, the current *DGA* abandoned previous guidelines' long-standing recommended limits on total fats.

The *DGA* recommends limiting saturated fat to less than 10 percent of your total calorie intake each day. Foods high in saturated fat include butter, cream, whole milk, cheeses, meats not labeled as "lean," and tropical oils such as palm oil and coconut oil. The *DGA* also continues to warn against trans fats found in processed food products that contain partially hydrogenated vegetable oils; these have largely been phased out, however.

What should you choose instead? Opt for healthier mono- and polyunsaturated fats, found in nuts, seeds, vegetable oils, avocados, and fatty fish.

Another change concerns dietary cholesterol, which was formerly emphasized as a key contributor to unhealthy levels of cholesterol in the blood. Saturated fat is a more significant contributor to unhealthy blood cholesterol levels than the cholesterol you consume from food. Experts now say healthy people don't need to avoid foods such as eggs and shrimp, which are high in dietary cholesterol but otherwise are good nutrient sources.

Avoid Added Sugars

Another concept gaining in currency among nutrition experts is the importance of avoiding "added sugars." That term refers to sugar in any form added to a food or beverage product, as opposed to naturally occurring sugars such as those in fruit and milk. While all sugar affects the body similarly, naturally occurring sugars come in combination with other nutrients like the vitamin C in fruit or the calcium in milk. Added sugars contribute only sweetness and calories.

The *DGA* advises limiting added sugars to less than 10 percent of calories per day. In a 2,000-calorie daily diet, that means no more than 200 calories from added sugars, which is roughly equivalent to 12 teaspoons or 52 grams of sugar—about the amount in one regular 16-ounce soft drink.

Identifying added sugars in foods and beverages can be tricky, since current Nutrition Facts labels are required to list only "total sugars." However, the U.S. Food and Drug Administration (FDA) has announced that revisions must be made to the Nutrition Facts label, which include listing both total sugars and added sugars. Some food manufacturers

---

Learn to Recognize the Many Names for Sugar

- Agave nectar
- Barley malt syrup
- Brown sugar
- Cane syrup
- Coconut sugar
- Corn sweetener
- Corn syrup
- Demerara sugar
- Dextrose
- Evaporated cane juice
- Fructose
- Fruit juice concentrate
- Glucose
- High-fructose corn syrup
- Honey
- Invert sugar
- Lactose
- Maltose
- Maple syrup
- Molasses
- Raw sugar
- Sucrose
- Syrup
- Table sugar

have revised their labels already, and the FDA is requiring all food manufacturers to make the revisions by January 2020 (January 2021 for smaller companies). If the food product you're considering doesn't list added sugars on the Nutrition Facts label, check the ingredients list for sugar, of which there are many types, including corn syrup, dextrose, molasses, and evaporated cane juice.

Watch the Salt

You're probably already watching your salt intake, especially if you're concerned about high blood pressure. Despite some controversy over the relative dangers of consuming too much sodium from salt, the DGA advises limiting sodium intake to less than 2,300 milligrams daily—the amount in about a teaspoon of ordinary iodized table salt.

Cut Down on Refined Grains

Adding to the advice to "make half your grains whole," the DGA calls for limiting intake of refined grains and products made with refined grains such as white flour. In addition, products made with refined flour, such as cookies, cakes, and many snack foods, often are high in other undesirable ingredients, including saturated fat, added sugars, and/or sodium.

Another area of emerging scientific interest is the downside of consuming too much refined starch, which is found in foods that are high in carbohydrates and lower in fiber. This may be addressed in the next DGA update; in the meantime, it's probably smart to limit starchy foods such as white potatoes (unless you also eat the fiber-rich skin) and other carb sources low in fiber.

Moderate Meat Consumption

A mounting body of evidence points to the association of many chronic diseases with diets high in red and processed meats. The scientific experts who advised the government about the current DGA

Striking a Balance with Carbs

When it comes to carbohydrates, the healthiest strategy seems to be a Goldilocks approach: not too much, but not too little, either. Evidence for "just right" carbohydrate intake comes from a meta-analysis of eight studies totaling more than 400,000 participants. A high-carb diet, with more than 70 percent of calories from carbohydrates, was associated with a 23 percent greater mortality risk. But a low-carb diet, with less than 40 percent of calories from carbohydrates, was associated with almost the same increase in mortality risk. The "just right" level for carb intake was seen in diets obtaining 50 to 55 percent of calories from carbohydrates. "Our findings suggest a U-shaped relationship between life expectancy and overall carbohydrate intake," the researchers concluded. In a smaller analysis of three studies, researchers found that mortality risk increased when people ate more animal protein in place of carbs, as in some popular diets. When plant-based proteins replaced carbs, however, mortality risk decreased.

The Lancet Public Health, August 16, 2018

recommended that people consume less red and processed meats. Those guidelines did not explicitly echo this advice, although they do emphasize eating a variety of protein-rich foods, including seafood and plant foods such as legumes, nuts, seeds, and soy products. Processed meats, such as sausage, ham, bacon, hot dogs, and cold cuts, also are sources of sodium and saturated fat, the DGA warns—and they have been classified as carcinogens, which are known to cause cancer. (Red meat has been classified as a probable carcinogen.)

Benefits of a Mediterranean Diet

The annual rankings of diets by *U.S. News and World Report* once again selected the Mediterranean diet as the healthiest, and the DGA specifically recommends this dietary pattern. The Mediterranean diet has been linked to reduced risks of heart disease, type 2 diabetes, obesity, some types of cancer, and cognitive decline.

Eating like a Mediterranean might even help you live longer. Research has found that older adults who ate more fruits, vegetables, and fish were less likely to die during a nine-year follow-up period than those who ate less of these foods. Fruits, vegetables, and fish are key components of the Mediterranean diet.

Eat Mediterranean to Live Longer

Following a Mediterranean-style dietary pattern has once again been associated with a longer life. Previous studies also have found this association, but this research, along with a meta-analysis of similar studies conducted by the authors, looked specifically at individuals ages 65 and older. The study analyzed data on 5,200 older adults for an average of eight years. Their diets were scored on a scale of 0 to 9 for how well they met criteria for a Mediterranean diet, with a score of 9 indicating that the diet met all the criteria. Higher diet scores were associated with a lower risk of death. In the meta-analysis, which pooled information from three studies totaling more than 11,500 participants, each one-point increase in diet score was associated with a 5 percent lower risk of dying during the study period.

British Journal of Nutrition, October 28, 2018

According to a study published in 2018 in the *Journal of the American Geriatrics Society*, adhering to a Mediterranean diet may help older individuals fend off frailty. Frailty, which is associated with a loss of muscle mass and greater vulnerability to issues arising with aging, predicts numerous negative health outcomes in older people, including falls, fractures, and hospitalizations. The analysis of four prior studies concluded that following a Mediterranean diet, especially emphasizing plant-based foods such as fruits and vegetables, whole grains, legumes, and nuts, was associated with a significantly lower risk of becoming frail. Overall, individuals with the highest Mediterranean diet scores were 56 percent less likely to develop frailty, compared to those with the lowest scores.

NEW FINDING

Mediterranean Diet Also Benefits Bones

The Mediterranean diet, already studied for heart and brain benefits, might also help protect bones in older women. A study of 103 healthy postmenopausal Brazilian women found that adherence to a Mediterranean-style eating pattern was associated with higher bone mineral density, specifically in the lumbar spine. Higher adherence also was associated with a greater appendicular lean mass index, a measure of lean muscle mass that can help ward off frailty. Researchers calculated diet scores based on the participants' intake of fruits, vegetables, legumes, cereals, fish, alcohol, olive oil, dairy, and meat. Higher intake of olive oil was most strongly associated with a lower percentage of body fat. "More studies are necessary to clarify the effect of Mediterranean diet on body composition," researchers concluded. "In the meantime, the emerging evidence suggests that the Mediterranean diet combined with other healthy lifestyle habits may be a useful non-pharmacological strategy for the primary prevention of osteoporosis and fractures in women after menopause."

Endocrine Society conference, March 2018

Mediterranean Diet Pyramid

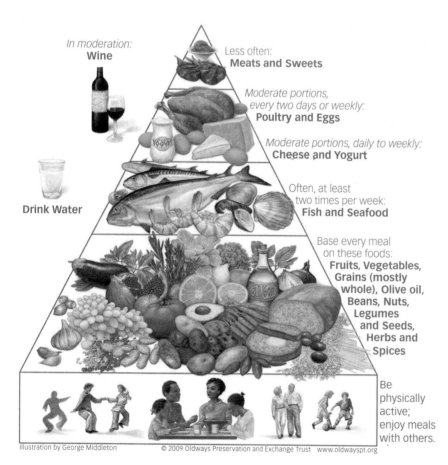

In moderation:
Wine

Less often:
Meats and Sweets

Moderate portions, every two days or weekly:
Poultry and Eggs

Moderate portions, daily to weekly:
Cheese and Yogurt

Drink Water

Often, at least two times per week:
Fish and Seafood

Base every meal on these foods:
Fruits, Vegetables, Grains (mostly whole), Olive oil, Beans, Nuts, Legumes and Seeds, Herbs and Spices

Be physically active; enjoy meals with others.

Illustration by George Middleton

© 2009 Oldways Preservation and Exchange Trust   www.oldwayspt.org

What Is a "Mediterranean" Diet?

So the evidence is strong that following a Mediterranean diet can benefit healthy aging. But what exactly does a "Mediterranean diet" mean? The truth is, there is no official Mediterranean diet the way there is an Atkins or South Beach diet.

The Mediterranean diet as tested in research studies includes many of the same key ingredients found in MyPlate for Older Adults. The chief difference between a Mediterranean-style diet and other healthy-eating plans (such as DASH, described next in this chapter) is the emphasis on unsaturated fats found in plant foods, especially monounsaturated fat in the form of olive oil.

But a "Mediterranean diet" does not include Italian meals piled with meatballs or sausage and rich sauces or pizza and sandwiches loaded with cheese and processed meats such as salami, pepperoni, and ham. The same goes for Greek specialties such as moussaka or spanakopita.

Instead, think of the foods traditionally consumed by working-class people in the Mediterranean region prior to the 1960s, when globalization began to change eating habits worldwide. Most people ate what they grew, raised, or caught, along with what was available at their local community markets, especially if they lived in rural areas. And, they cooked meals at home and dined with family and friends; they didn't have the option of picking up dinner at a drive-through window.

One way to envision such a diet is to look at the "Mediterranean diet pyramid." At the bottom of the pyramid are the foods consumed most often, including fruits and vegetables, beans, nuts, healthy grains, and olive oil—all plant foods that are rich in a variety of nutrients. Animal-sourced foods eaten most frequently include fish and seafood. The foods eaten least often are meats and sweets, followed by poultry, eggs, cheese, and yogurt—foods that tend to be high in saturated fat and, in the case of sweets, added sugar.

Mediterranean at the Supermarket

Switching to a Mediterranean diet starts with rethinking your supermarket route, especially if you typically head for the packaged-foods aisles. Grocery shopping for a Mediterranean diet can be easily done in most stores if you go prepared with a little knowledge and a plan. Here's a basic section-by-section strategy:

▶ **Produce section:** A Mediterranean diet stresses whole and fresh foods, so the produce section is the best place to start. Stock up on seasonal fruits and vegetables to create the backbone of your diet. Fruit also can be your go-to choice for desserts.

▶ **Meat and fish counter:** Here's where your grocery cart will really start to look different. Despite the current diet craze of low-carb eating and high meat intake, a traditional Mediterranean diet goes light on meat and focuses instead on plant foods. When you're eating less red meat, you'll want to boost your consumption of seafood. Fish high in heart-healthy omega-3 fatty acids such as salmon are excellent choices. The easiest way to go more Mediterranean is to substitute seafood (baked, broiled, or steamed, not fried) for meat.

▶ **Dry goods:** Eating like a Mediterranean doesn't mean giving up the convenience of canned and packaged foods, as long as you pick carefully. Dried beans and other legumes are an economical choice, but canned, low-sodium options are okay, too—just make sure to drain and rinse to further reduce sodium. Canned tomatoes make it easy to jump-start a Mediterranean-style meal. Choose whole-grain pastas, brown rice, and other whole-grain products.

▶ **Oils:** Use olive oil instead of butter for cooking.

▶ **Snacks and sweets:** Skip the candy and cookies aisles except for special treats. Substitute unsalted nuts—whatever variety you prefer—and seeds such as sunflower or pumpkin for chips and other snacks.

▶ **Dairy case:** Dairy is not a huge component of the Mediterranean diet, although you can enjoy plain, unsweetened dairy products. Sweeten your yogurt with fruit, for example, and sprinkle on the cheese instead of adding it by the handful.

▶ **Beverage aisle:** Sugary sodas are definitely not part of the traditional Mediterranean diet. Water is your best choice, though you also can drink wine with meals in moderation.

DASH to Beat Hypertension

Tying the Mediterranean diet in the previous year's rankings, the Dietary Approaches to Stop Hypertension (DASH) plan was designed by the National Heart, Lung and Blood Institute. This eating plan is based on findings from large clinical studies that tested the effects of sodium and other nutrients on blood pressure. Hypertension—high blood pressure—is a key risk factor for cardiovascular disease and stroke. Following a healthy diet based on whole foods will help keep

Eating for Brain Health

Researchers in Australia report further evidence of benefits from the MIND diet, a hybrid of the Mediterranean and DASH diets that focuses on brain health. Over a follow-up period of 12 years, greater adherence to the MIND diet was associated with a 19 percent lower risk of cognitive impairment, Alzheimer's disease, and other dementias, according to the study of 1,220 adults, ages 60 and older. By contrast, no similar benefit was seen for sticking to a Mediterranean diet without the specific brain-health emphases of the MIND plan, such as eating berries twice a week and leafy greens six times a week. The data came from a study in which participants initially completed questionnaires about their diets and then were assessed for cognitive abilities and impairment over time. Their diets were scored for greater or lesser adherence to the MIND and Mediterranean diet patterns.

Alzheimer's & Dementia, April 2019

your intake of sodium and potassium in balance, which will improve your blood pressure and reduce your risk of disease. Study results showed that the greatest blood pressure reduction occurred with a DASH plan that was lowest in sodium— just 1,500 milligrams daily.

But eating the DASH way isn't just good for your blood pressure. Even if you have no worries about hypertension, DASH provides an easy-to-follow model of overall healthy eating. In a review of six studies that examined the DASH-style diet in relation to heart health, researchers linked this dietary pattern to a 20 percent reduction in cardiovascular disease, a 21 percent reduction in coronary heart disease, a 19 percent reduction in stroke, and a 29 percent reduction in heart failure.

Here are some steps to get you started:

Eat More
- Fruits
- Vegetables
- Whole grains
- Nuts and legumes
- Low-fat dairy (2–3 daily servings)

Eat Less
- Red and processed meats
- Sweetened beverages
- Sodium

You can download the complete DASH plan for free at https://bit.ly/2DwM8pe.

Your Brain on the MIND Diet

Another dietary pattern that's been making headlines, the Mediterranean-DASH Intervention for Neurogenerative Delay, seems like quite a mouthful until you understand its acronym: MIND. This newer regimen, focused on dementia prevention and memory protection, combines aspects of both the Mediterranean and DASH diets, along with the latest findings about nutrition and the brain. The MIND diet emphasizes "natural, plant-based foods and limited intakes of animal and high saturated-fat

foods, but uniquely specifies the consumption of berries and green leafy vegetables," according to researchers who developed the diet.

Though the MIND diet was specifically studied for the effects it had on brain health and function, it embodies many of the principles of healthy eating we've seen in other patterns. It includes at least three servings of whole grains, a serving of leafy green vegetables, and one other vegetable every day. It also calls for getting five or more servings of nuts each week and eating beans four or more times a week, poultry and berries at least twice a week, and fish at least once a week. The MIND diet recommends using olive oil as your main cooking oil. It allows up to one glass of wine per day.

On the other hand, the MIND diet identifies these five less-healthy food groups to limit:
- Red meat (no more than three servings a week)
- Butter and stick margarine (less than one tablespoon daily)
- Cheese (less than once per week)
- Pastries and sweets (no more than four times a week)
- Fried or fast food (less than once per week)

Benefits that have been associated with the MIND diet include a slower rate of cognitive decline and a lower risk of developing Alzheimer's disease.

Patterns for Life

Whether you follow one of these eating plans or create your own healthy eating pattern based on the information included in this book, you can start making a difference in your diet—and in your health—right away. The many benefits associated with the Mediterranean-style, DASH, and MIND dietary patterns provide powerful evidence that dietary changes can improve your quality of life and reduce your risk of life-threatening diseases as you grow older.

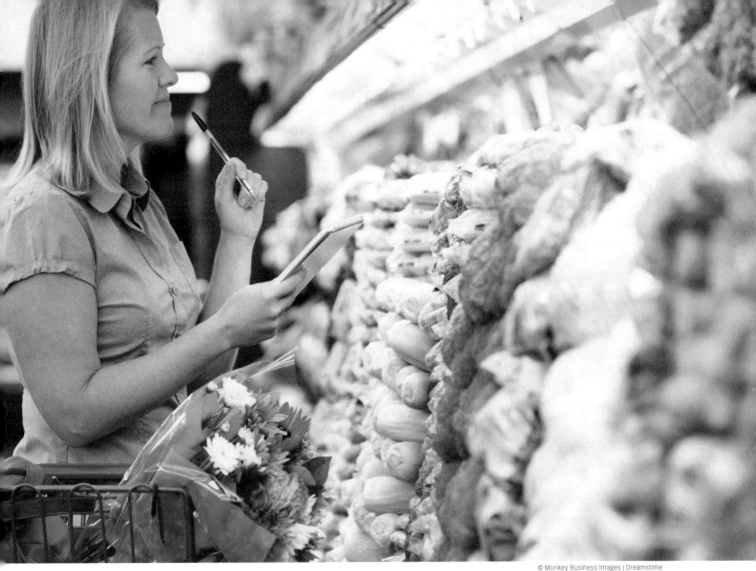

A healthy diet starts in the supermarket; making a shopping list can help you stick to smart choices and resist impulse buys.

3 Tasty, Affordable Nutrition

Even if you're convinced that adopting a healthier dietary pattern can help protect you as you age, you might still be thinking that eating right means eating boring food. Or you may be concerned that you can't afford to improve your diet. These are common misconceptions.

"We are beginning to have an adversarial relationship with food," says Alice H. Lichtenstein, DSc, director of Tufts' HNRCA Cardiovascular Nutrition Laboratory and co-creator of MyPlate for Older Adults. "We need to eat to live, to consume certain foods to meet our nutrient requirements. There are many ways of doing that, and you should be able to eat foods that you really enjoy while optimizing health outcomes and maintaining a healthy body weight."

Know Your Food Facts

You might even feel that simple grocery shopping has become a daunting task because of all the types of foods you've heard should be avoided. For example, some people think it's important to buy cage-free eggs, grass-fed beef, and wild-caught fish, or to buy foods that don't contain any genetically modified (GMO) ingredients (despite the weight of scientific evidence that these foods are safe). You've probably heard that it's best to reduce your intake of artificial colors, preservatives, and other additives—although no additives currently in the food supply have been definitively shown to present a hazard.

Add up all of these concerns, along with advice to avoid unhealthy fats, added sugars, and sodium, and it becomes challenging to feel good instead of guilty about eating.

Start with a reality check about what foods do and don't provide. "You shouldn't expect that each food will provide all the nutrients you need," says Dr. Lichtenstein. "You can't get your protein from fruits or your vitamin C from fish; it's the combinations that are important."

You can simplify your shopping by filling your grocery cart with whole and minimally processed foods. Since these foods have undergone few, if any, modifications, they don't contain a long list of ingredients you'll often find in heavily processed food products, such as salt, sugar, added fat, and additives. Whole, fresh foods don't have any ingredients lists because there are no added ingredients.

Don't Skip the Spices

MyPlate for Older Adults emphasizes spices as way to make healthy foods tastier. Research suggests that some spices might even trick your brain into liking less-salty foods. A large study in China reported that people with a penchant for spicier foods preferred less salt, which was associated with less sodium consumed overall and lower blood pressures. The results imply (but do not prove) that people who eat relatively spicy foods prefer less salt to satisfy their tastes—and vice versa.

Researchers further explored the connection using functional brain scanning. They scanned the brains of 60 volunteers, measuring activity in two regions of the brain involved in salt perception. The participants tasted salty water at two concentrations, with and without a bit of capsaicin (the compound that makes peppers hot)—though not enough to cause a burning sensation on the tongue. People who got capsaicin preferred the less-salty water. Moreover, the two brain regions associated with salt taste preferences were not as active when participants were given salty water with capsaicin, compared with people who just got salty water.

Eat Right on a Budget

Another misconception about healthy food is that it always costs more. You might think that eating a nutritious diet, especially one with lots of fruits and vegetables, must be more expensive than the typical American fare that includes packaged, processed, and fast foods. The good news is that eating right doesn't have to mean spending more money.

"Healthy food is not necessarily expensive," says Parke Wilde, PhD, an associate professor at Tufts' Friedman School who previously worked for the USDA's Economic Research Service. "It is true that some healthy food is high-priced, but many other healthy options are both tasty and affordable."

Dr. Wilde cites a USDA report that identified six changes that could improve consumers' diet quality; of the changes, none cost more, and most actually cost less, with savings up to $1.19 a day. The greatest cost savings and dietary improvement came from substituting a table-service restaurant meal with one prepared at home, along with switching from fast-food fare to home cooking. Another change that paid off as much as eating at home more often was skipping weekend splurges. Eating the same on Friday through Sunday as on weekdays saved money—and it improved consumers' scores on an index of healthy eating.

None of those changes will break your budget. In fact, making more meals at home from whole, unprocessed ingredients will save you money.

Find Your Pattern

Focusing on dietary patterns such as those we looked at in the previous chapter rather than on individual foods is one tasty way to change your thinking about healthy food choices. "The emphasis on dietary patterns reflects a shift from more prescriptive nutrition recommendations to more general ones," Dr. Lichtenstein says. "It provides flexibility to customize our everyday dietary patterns to foods that are both healthy and enjoyable. What works for one person does not necessarily work for someone else. The worst thing to happen is arguing over whether blueberries are better for you than raspberries, or canola oil is better than corn oil."

The Mediterranean diet, for example, has gained popularity not only because of research linking it to positive outcomes but also because it's fairly easy to follow—and it tastes good. It includes many foods people actually enjoy: a nice piece of fish, a handful of nuts, vegetables sautéed in olive oil, and even alcohol in moderation.

Other dietary patterns also can satisfy your palate while meeting your nutritional needs. Real Chinese food—as opposed to Chinese-American restaurant fare—leans heavily on vegetables, with minimal portions of poultry, seafood, or meat. Substitute brown rice for the refined white rice with your vegetable-laden moo goo gai pan or kung pao chicken, serve the sauce on the side, and you have a healthy meal that's also delicious. Similarly, authentic Mexican fare—not the cheese-laden, fast-food, Tex-Mex version—emphasizes beans, avocados, tomatoes, seafood, and other mostly healthy choices with a spicy kick that makes otherwise bland foods more appealing.

The Power of Portions

Whatever dietary pattern you prefer, don't overdo it; it's possible to eat too much, even if your food is healthy. Taking the time to savor your food can help control how much you eat, as can simply putting less food on your plate. Here are some tips for controlling portion size:

- **Use smaller plates,** bowls, and serving spoons. A plate nine inches in diameter is appropriate for lunch and dinner.
- **Avoid eating straight from the package.** If you're dipping directly into a box or bag, you won't know how much you've eaten.
- **For foods you eat regularly,** such as cold cereal or nuts, keep an inexpensive measuring cup or measuring spoon in or with the container so you can easily dish up an appropriate portion.
- **At a restaurant,** choose the smallest size available. If meals are oversized, put half in a to-go box as soon as you get your food or plan in advance to split your dish with a friend.
- **At home,** dish up a single serving at mealtime and leave extra portions in the kitchen. For snacks, fill reusable containers with single-serve portions from a bigger package.
- **Look for recipes that include nutrition information** and the number of servings.
- **Especially watch portion sizes of starch- and sugar-rich foods,** such as white bread, white rice, crackers, sweets, soda, sports drinks, and fruit juice, as well as alcohol, which are all easy to overdo and linked to weight gain.
- **Opt for nutrient-rich, minimally processed foods,** such as whole fruits, non-starchy vegetables, legumes (beans), nuts, and unsweetened low-fat or nonfat yogurt, which can more naturally help fill you up and help you manage your weight.

Helpful Kitchen Strategies

You can make it easier to choose tasty, affordable foods every day by having a variety of healthy choices in your pantry and fridge. With healthy options on hand, you'll be less tempted to eat junk food or run to the nearest fast-food place when hunger strikes. Here are some examples of items to keep in your pantry, fridge, and freezer.

NEW FINDING

Change Your Portion Perspective

Seeing smaller portions actually can create a "new normal," British researchers report. They found that reducing food portion sizes may shift a person's perceptions of what is a normal amount of food to eat and induce them to choose smaller portions next time. The researchers conducted a series of three experiments. In the first experiment, female diners were randomly assigned to receive one of two portions (large or small) of quiche for lunch. The next day, the participants returned and were invited to serve themselves whatever portion they desired; those who had been served the smaller portion the day before tended to choose smaller portions. The second experiment was identical to the first, except the participants were male, and produced the same results. In the third experiment, both male and female diners were assessed a week after the initial lunch. Researchers administered a visual questionnaire to gauge what portion sizes looked "normal" to the participants. Diners previously served smaller portions rated the smaller portions on the questionnaire as more normal.
American Journal of Clinical Nutrition, April 2018

In the Pantry or Cupboards

- Whole-grain pastas
- Instant, quick-cooking, or microwaveable brown rice and other whole grains
- Whole-wheat flour
- Canned vegetables (choose low-sodium varieties)
- Reduced-sodium tomato sauce
- Canned beans (drain and rinse before using)
- Canned fruits in juice (no added sugars)
- Dried fruits
- Unsalted or low-salt nuts and seeds
- Peanut butter or other nut butters, preferably the "natural" type with little to no sugar, oil, or salt added
- Reduced-sodium chicken and vegetable broth (refrigerate after opening)
- Canned (in water) or pouch-packed fish, such as salmon, sardines, and tuna
- Vinegars to use in homemade salad dressings
- Dried herbs and spices, pepper, and low-sodium seasoning blends
- Powdered egg whites
- Popcorn (kernels, not microwavable packages that contain added fats and salt)
- Whole-grain sandwich breads, "thins," pita bread, and crackers
- Whole-grain, high-fiber, low-sugar cereals and oatmeal
- Onions, garlic, and sweet potatoes (store in a cool, dark pantry)
- Oils high in unsaturated fat, such as olive, canola, soybean, and corn oils
- Cooking oil spray

In the Refrigerator

- Fat-free or low-fat milk, yogurt, cheese, and cottage cheese
- Plain, unsweetened non-dairy "milk" (almond, soy, cashew, etc.)
- Fruits and vegetables with a relatively long shelf life (e.g., apples, carrots, grapes)
- Light "buttery" vegetable-oil spread that contains no partially hydrogenated oil
- Eggs/egg substitutes
- Whole-wheat flour tortillas
- Low-sodium condiments such as mustard, salsa, and hot sauce
- Salad dressings low in sodium and added sugar
- Lemons and limes or lemon and lime juice

In the Freezer

- Frozen vegetables and vegetable mixes (no added salt or sauces)
- Frozen berries (no added sugar)
- Pre-portioned seafood, lean meats, ground turkey, and boneless, skinless chicken breasts and thighs

Supplement these staples on your supermarket shopping trips by purchasing an assortment of perishable produce, such as salad greens, peppers, tomatoes, fresh berries, bananas, and melons.

"Processed" Foods: Pros and Cons

Often, eating more healthfully is seen as synonymous with avoiding all processed foods, but that's not necessarily the case; it depends on the degree of processing. The U.S. government defines "processed food" as "any food other than a raw agricultural commodity that has been subject to processing, such as canning, cooking, freezing, dehydration, or milling." There are varying degrees of processing; many highly processed foods contain added salt, sugar, fat, additives, and other ingredients that contribute nothing in terms of nutrition.

But that doesn't mean all "processed" food is automatically bad. Many minimally processed foods provide plenty of valuable nutrients, are more convenient, and reduce the risk of foodborne illness. Minimally processed foods include:

- Pasteurized milk
- Prewashed lettuce and spinach
- Canned beans, vegetables, and fruits
- "Baby" carrots
- Oatmeal
- Frozen and canned fish
- Whole-grain flours
- Frozen fruits and vegetables
- Yogurt

"You hear the term 'processed food' thrown around a lot these days, but you have to use common sense," says Tufts' Dr. Lichtenstein. "For example, pasteurized milk is safer than unpasteurized, even though, technically, it is 'processed.'"

Some forms of processing actually boost the nutrition you'll get from certain foods. For example, cutting and chopping produce can make nutrients more available to your body by doing some of the work of breaking down cell walls. So can heating, including the heat of canning: The lycopene in canned tomatoes and tomato sauces is more accessible than in fresh, uncooked tomatoes. However, heat depletes some other vitamins, such as vitamin C and some B vitamins.

And, when you consider food costs, both in dollars and in preparation time, research indicates that using minimally processed foods is less costly.

Frozen vs. Fresh

Another form of processing that there's no need to avoid is freezing. Freezing makes seafood more readily available, for example. Unless you live near a coast, frozen seafood can be the best way to meet recommendations to eat fish twice a week. Shop for flash-frozen fish labeled "Frozen-at-Sea" (FAS), caught by ships that operate like floating processing plants. Each day's catch is processed, frozen in a matter of seconds,

and stored at zero degrees or below. The result is fish that's often fresher than what's sold as "fresh," which might be kept on ice for as long as two weeks between ship and supermarket.

Produce is another smart choice in the frozen-food aisle. Research has confirmed that frozen produce is at least as nutritious as fresh, and certain nutrients are better preserved in frozen vegetables and fruits than in fresh produce after a few days in your fridge. In as little as five days, fresh produce loses some of its vitamin content, especially vitamins A and C and folate.

Think of freezing as "nature's pause button." Freezing foods maintains freshness, slows down enzymatic reactions, and increases the time it takes the food to degrade. Fresh produce, by contrast, is a living material, with oxidation and enzyme activity. It degrades over time and loses nutrients.

Not everything about frozen veggies "pauses" perfectly, of course. Texture can suffer when vegetables are frozen, such as with bell peppers or green beans, even if the nutrients mostly survive intact. As a result, you're better off incorporating some frozen vegetables into stews, soups, and other mixed dishes. Other vegetables freeze with little loss of texture, such as peas, lima beans, and corn, and can be as appealing (and easier to prepare) as fresh.

Dr. Lichtenstein adds, "When buying frozen vegetables and fruits, an easy rule is to get the item only and nothing else; that means skipping the sauces and seasonings." When in doubt, check the package for the ingredients; it should show only the name of the food (for example, spinach or strawberries), with no other added ingredients.

Processed Meat Cautions

When applied to meats, however, the term "processed" has a very distinct meaning. The American Institute for

Frozen Fish Tips

When shopping for frozen fish, keep these tips in mind:

- Dig deep down in the freezer case for rock-hard fish with package dates no more than three months old.
- Avoid packages that are positioned above the "frost line" or top of the freezer case.
- Avoid frozen seafood if the package is open, torn, or crushed on the edges, and don't buy packages with signs of frost or ice crystals, which may mean the fish has been stored a long time or thawed and refrozen.

To thaw frozen fish for cooking, set unopened packages in the refrigerator the previous day; if pressed for time, thaw in a bowl of cold water on the counter, changing the water several times.

Cancer Research (AICR) defines processed meat as "meat preserved by smoking, curing or salting, or addition of chemical preservatives," and says that even small amounts eaten regularly increase the risk of colorectal cancer. The World Health Organization (WHO) also has announced that foods such as hot dogs, ham, bacon, sausages, and deli meats contribute to the risk of colon, stomach, and other cancers.

According to the WHO, about 34,000 cancer deaths per year worldwide are attributable to diets high in processed meats. While that number pales in comparison to the 1 million or so global cancer deaths related to smoking, it is significant enough to warrant a hard look at processed meats in your diet, especially because they also are associated with cardiovascular disease and other health conditions.

What counts as "processed meat"? Bacon, sausages, hot dogs, jerky, salami, pepperoni, and cold cuts like bologna, ham, or smoked turkey are examples of processed meat. Scientists believe that chemicals added to meat during processing may be responsible for the increased cancer risk, but a cause-and-effect relationship has not been conclusively established.

Nitrates and Nitrites. Sodium nitrite and sodium nitrate (which naturally converts to sodium nitrite) are used as preservatives in processed meats because they prevent bacterial growth. Nitrates also are found naturally in a number of foods, including celery, beets, arugula, and other vegetables. "It is common nowadays to find the statement 'no added nitrates' on processed meat products," says Joel B. Mason, MD, professor of medicine and nutrition at Tufts and director of the HNRCA Vitamins and Carcinogenesis Laboratory. "In most instances, these products are manufactured using celery juice or other natural sources of nitrates."

But don't be fooled by this labeling. Dr. Mason cautions that there is no evidence that the nitrates in celery juice act any differently in the body than nitrates added as food-grade chemicals. "In fact, unlike food-grade sodium nitrate or nitrite, there is no federal regulation

Processed Meat and Cancer

Is the slice of bacon on your BLT really as dangerous as smoking a cigarette? That was the implication of some of the scary headlines based on a World Health Organization (WHO) report stating that processed meat is a carcinogen that raises the risk of colon, stomach, and other cancers.

The WHO's listing of processed meat such as bacon and cold cuts as a "Group 1" carcinogen—the same group that contains smoking and asbestos—doesn't mean it's equally dangerous. Rather, the designation reflects the strength of the evidence linking processed meats to cancer risk.

The connection between meats and cancer risk should come as no surprise. Joel B. Mason, MD, director of Tufts' HNRCA Vitamins and Carcinogenesis Laboratory, comments, "The only change that occurred from my perspective is that the WHO finally codified the previously known link between cancer and red/processed meat into a report."

How much is too much? The WHO report said there aren't enough data to define how much processed meat is dangerous, but the data do show that risk increases with consumption. An analysis of 10 studies indicated that eating about 1.75 ounces of processed meat daily was associated with an added lifetime risk of colorectal cancer of roughly 18 percent. That's about the equivalent of one hot dog or a couple of slices of cold cuts or bacon.

Limiting Your Risk

How can you reduce your risk? Since it's not clear what kinds of "processing" cause processed meats to be more carcinogenic, simply choosing nitrate-free meats may not reduce your risk. The American Institute for Cancer Research does offer some ideas for cutting processed-meat consumption:

- Replace packaged deli meats with freshly cooked, sliced chicken or turkey or canned tuna (in water, not oil).

- Try spicy vegetarian sausages instead of bacon, chorizo, or salami.

- Replace sausage in chili and sauces with legumes such as kidney beans, chickpeas, and lentils.

- Use herbs and spices such as garlic, fennel seed, and hot pepper flakes to add flavor in place of processed meats.

that limits how much celery juice can be added to a processed meat, so it is feasible to actually be consuming more nitrates with a processed meat that says, 'no added nitrates'."

When consumed in vegetables, nitrates are safe, and may even have protective health effects such as improving blood flow. But in meats, nitrites can react during processing, cooking, and storage to form compounds called nitrosamines, which are classified as carcinogens. "Keep in mind, however, that the link between sodium nitrate and cancer risk is still unclear," says Dr. Mason.

Healthy, Satisfying Snacks

When planning your healthy dietary pattern, don't overlook snacks. Between-meal foods and beverages now total a quarter of Americans' average daily calorie intake—amounting to what researchers call a "full eating event." Eating healthier meals won't improve your overall diet if you grab high-calorie, nutrient-poor foods at snack time.

Everything a person eats and drinks contributes to their overall dietary pattern. "Snacks should fit into total dietary intake for the day," says Helen Rasmussen, PhD, RD, a senior research dietitian at Tufts' Jean Mayer USDA Human Nutrition Research Center on Aging and co-developer of MyPlate for Older Adults.

Shifting away from thinking of daily snacks as treats or extras to seeing them in their rightful place as part of the overall dietary pattern can help you make choices that contribute to the quality of your diet, rather than detracting from it. "People should choose snacks that fill holes in their diet," says Dr. Lichtenstein. "For some people it's dairy, for some fruit and vegetables or whole grains."

So healthy snack foods should meet the same standards you set for mealtime

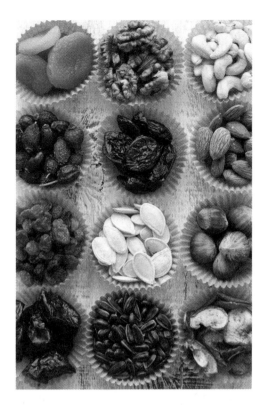

© Alena Ozerova | Dreamstime

Portion out snack foods before you begin eating to reduce the chance of overeating.

choices. Pick foods that are nutrient-dense—delivering plenty of nutrition per calorie—and select whole, minimally processed snacks over refined products high in added sugars and sodium. Go for whole grains and high-fiber snacks, which will satisfy your hunger longer between meals.

Snack Survival Tips

Keep these tips in mind when reaching for between-meal bites:

▶ **Plan ahead to have healthy snacks** like washed and cut-up fruits and vegetables, yogurt, hard-boiled eggs, whole grain crackers, cheeses, nuts and nut butters, hummus, and air-popped popcorn on hand.

▶ **Portion out snacks.** Research has found that people consistently consume more food and drink when offered larger-sized portions or packages than when offered smaller-sized versions. Portion out foods ahead of time for grab-and-go snacking, and use smaller bowls and plates.

▶ **Deal with boredom and stress.** Eating out of boredom or for emotional reasons can lead to overeating. Stop and rate your true hunger level before reaching for a snack.

- **Eat mindfully.** Eat slowly and pay attention to fullness cues to avoid mindless eating.
- **Avoid temptation.** Notice when you're in a setting or situation with unhealthy snacks. Change your route to avoid a habitual stop at the doughnut shop, and move the office candy jar out of sight or out of reach.
- **Don't be fooled by labeling.** In one study, women who had eaten pasta labeled as a "snack" later ate significantly more candy than women who were given the same pasta serving labeled as a "meal." Trust visual clues or the body's hunger/satiety cues, not the package label.
- **Sit down.** The same study found that participants who stood and ate their pasta from a container consumed more sweets in a follow-up taste test than those who sat and ate the pasta from a plate. Distracted eating (like eating in front of the television or while reading or working) also may lead to increased food intake.
- **Practice food safety.** When carrying snacks, keep perishable foods refrigerated or in a cooler bag with ice packs.
- **Remember it's optional.** While snacking is appropriate for some people, it is not a mandatory part of a healthy eating pattern.

Finally, avoid wasting valuable calories on sodas or other sweet drinks. For between-meal beverages, choose low-sodium tomato or mixed vegetable juices, unsweetened iced tea, fat-free milk, or low-or no-calorie flavored sparkling or seltzer water.

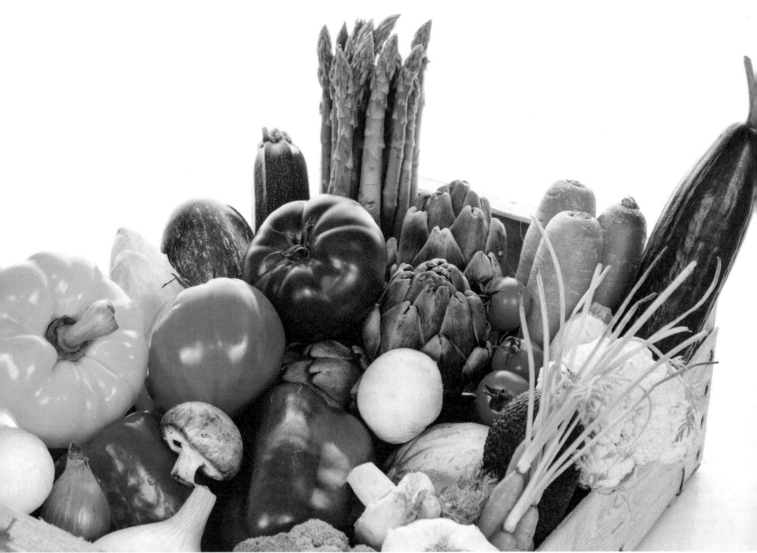

Vegetables are excellent sources of vitamins and minerals, fiber, and micronutrients that have health benefits.

4 Vegetable "Superfoods"

You can hardly walk into a grocery store, peruse a newsstand, or turn on a TV health program without being bombarded by claims for "superfoods." Scientifically, that term is meaningless hype, but practically, if you're trying to eat more so-called "superfoods," you can start by consuming more vegetables—of almost any type. Diane L. McKay, PhD, a professor and researcher at Tufts and the Tufts consulting editor for this report, explains: "They're all super! Eating a variety of vegetables and other healthy foods is the basis of a good diet. There isn't any one whole food that will meet all of your nutrition requirements."

In all of the various rating systems for foods, she adds, certain groups of foods always come out on top—those that are plant-based. Vegetables are excellent sources of fiber, as well as many of the nutrients you may need more of as you age. The health benefits are clear: People who consume more plant-based foods, including vegetables, fruits, and whole grains, have a lower risk of cardiovascular disease and certain cancers.

Not surprisingly, on the Tufts' MyPlate for Older Adults, vegetables occupy more space than any other food group.

Five-a-Day Is Just a Start

You've probably also heard that eating five servings a day of vegetables and fruits is a healthy goal. According to research published in the *International*

Eat Your Veggies to Fight Breast Cancer

Cruciferous vegetables and yellow-orange veggies seem to be especially effective in lowering the risk for invasive breast cancer. Researchers looked at the diets of 182,145 women over an average of 24 years, during which 10,911 cases of invasive breast cancer were diagnosed. Compared with eating less than two-and-a-half servings (about a cup) of fruits and vegetables daily, consuming at least five-and-a-half servings was associated with an 11 percent lower breast cancer incidence. The produce most strongly associated with lower risk included cruciferous vegetables like cauliflower, Brussels sprouts, and kale, as well as yellow-orange vegetables such as carrots, winter squash, yams, and sweet potatoes.

International Journal of Cancer,
July 6, 2018

Journal of Epidemiology, however, that's just a good start. The analysis of 95 observational studies concluded that eating five servings of vegetables and fruits daily was associated with a 14 percent lower risk of heart disease, while eating 10 servings a day was associated with a 24 percent lower risk, compared to zero servings. (A serving is one-half cup cooked vegetables or a small piece of fruit.)

The researchers commented, "If you can't fit in 10 servings of fruits and vegetables, it may be worthwhile to at least make sure you eat some of the specific ones we found were associated with reduced heart disease risk," such as leafy greens, cruciferous vegetables (broccoli, cauliflower, Brussels sprouts, and cabbage), citrus fruits, apples, and pears.

Lesser-Known Nutrients

What makes vegetables so good for you? Most are excellent sources of essential vitamins and minerals, along with fiber. But some of the health benefits of vegetables (as well as fruits) also can be attributed to lesser-known natural plant compounds called phytonutrients (also referred to as "phytochemicals"). Phytonutrients help protect plants from bugs, fungi, and infections. Phytonutrients often are found in the highest amounts in vegetables' outer surfaces or peels, and usually, they are responsible for the pigments that give many vegetables their distinctive colors.

"Phytonutrients are not classic nutrients like vitamins," says Dr. McKay. "These are compounds that several studies have shown have biological activity that confers health benefits, such as improving markers of chronic disease risk. Nearly all phytonutrients have antioxidant activity, but that is not necessarily their mode of action in the body. Within cells, they may turn signals on or off, reduce inflammation, or trigger a whole cascade of events."

Types of phytonutrients include carotenoids (found in carrots, winter squash, tomatoes, and yellow peppers), organo sulfides (found in onions, garlic, broccoli, and cabbage), and phytosterols (found in peas, soybeans, and vegetable oils).

There are no minimum daily requirements for the more than 25,000 phytonutrients that scientists have identified in plants. These compounds are not essential to keeping you alive the way that, say, protein, carbohydrates, water, or vitamins are. Many of the health benefits of phytonutrients, which also are found in tea, coffee, cocoa, whole grains, and fruits, are still being studied. "Thousands of different phytonutrients have been identified to date, and we're still going," Dr. McKay says.

Some research suggests phytonutrients in vegetables and fruits might help protect against some forms of cancer. For example, eating foods containing beta-cryptoxanthin (BCX)—a red pigment abundant in sweet red peppers, paprika, winter squash, oranges, and tangerines, among other foods—might work at the molecular level to thwart lung cancer. And a dietary pattern high in colorful vegetables and fruits, such as carrots, pumpkin, sweet potatoes, peppers, cantaloupe, and dark leafy greens, seems to help protect against breast cancer.

A Variety of Phytonutrients

One reason to consume a wide mix of plant foods in your diet is to obtain a variety of phytonutrients. "Each plant food provides a different array of phytonutrients that work together synergistically," Dr. McKay says.

The combinations of phytonutrients found in plant foods produce greater benefits than you'd get if you were to isolate the individual nutrients and then take them together. The many nutrients present in whole foods are uniquely balanced, and they produce an effect greater than any effect you can get by taking nutrients in supplement form. This is one reason why nutrition experts advise getting nutrients from whole foods rather than supplements.

Trending Vegetarian

You don't have to become a vegetarian to eat more veggies, but studies of vegetarians do provide convincing evidence of the health benefits of eating more plant-based foods. In one such study, vegetarians were 32 percent less likely to suffer coronary artery disease than non-vegetarians. The benefits were seen in participants who had been following a vegetarian diet for less than five years, as well as in long-term vegetarians. Other research has found that vegetarians tend to have lower risks of heart disease, certain cancers, diabetes, obesity, and hypertension.

The health benefits of vegetables and other plant foods and/or concerns about animal welfare and the environment lead some people to choose a vegetarian dietary pattern. Vegetarian diets are becoming more mainstream, and the 2015-2020 *Dietary Guidelines for Americans* includes a vegetarian eating pattern as one of its three examples of healthy diet plans.

Another healthy option is to limit or give up meat but keep seafood on the menu: Other research suggests that a pescatarian diet—one that includes fish as well as an abundance of plant foods—might be even more healthful than a strict vegetarian regimen. One report showed that people who are otherwise vegetarians but eat fish at least once a month had the lowest incidence of colorectal cancer. Adding fish to a vegetarian diet was associated with less risk than any other type of vegetarian diet, including a vegan regimen, which includes no dairy, eggs, fish, or animal products of any kind.

You can follow a plant-based diet even if you're not a vegetarian; it's not an all-or-nothing choice. There's no ironclad definition for the term "plant-based diet"; generally, it means that the majority of foods eaten are from plant rather than animal sources. If your diet includes several servings of animal proteins each day, chances are you're not getting enough fruits, vegetables, and whole grains. It would be a healthy move to eat more plant-based foods and fewer animal-sourced foods, even if you're not giving up beef, pork, or poultry completely.

Moreover, following a vegetarian diet doesn't guarantee that the diet is healthy; it all depends on which plant-based foods you choose. "Fries and a Coke are vegetarian," says Dariush Mozaffarian, MD, DrPH, dean of Tufts' Friedman School of Nutrition Science and Policy. "More important than what you avoid is what you actually eat. The healthiest diets are rich in fruits, nuts, fish, vegetables, yogurt, beans, vegetable oils, and whole grains. Being or not being a vegetarian does not add much to that."

Boosting Your Veggies

Whatever dietary pattern you choose, you'll want to put lots of veggies in your shopping cart. You can find nutritious vegetable options in the produce section, the frozen foods case, and even the canned goods aisle. To be a smart vegetable consumer, keep these tips in mind:

▶ **Buy fresh vegetables in season,** adapting your menus to match the harvest. In-season vegetables will be cheaper and are likely to be at their peak of flavor and nutrients.

▶ **Keep frozen vegetables handy** in your freezer to quickly heat up in the microwave as a side dish or to add to soups, stews, and casseroles. (Remember that frozen veggies are at least as nutritious as fresh.)

▶ **Pay a little more for convenience if it means you'll eat more veggies.** Pick up pre-washed bags of salad greens,

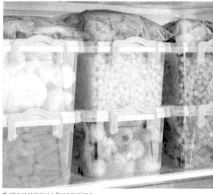
© Chernetskaya | Dreamstime

Keep frozen vegetables on hand; you can pull them out and serve them in a matter of minutes.

Vegetables Highest and Lowest in Pesticides

Choosing organic vegetables can minimize the amount of pesticides you consume. The Environmental Working Group (www.ewg.org) annually tests and rates produce for pesticide residue. These vegetables, which ranked in the EWG's latest "Dirty Dozen," are the most likely to contain pesticides and are the most important to buy organic if that's a concern:

- Spinach
- Celery
- Kale
- Potatoes
- Tomatoes

Conventionally grown veggies that are listed in the EWG's "Clean Fifteen" of produce with the least pesticides include:

- Avocados
- Sweet Corn
- Sweet peas (frozen)
- Onions
- Eggplant
- Asparagus
- Cabbage
- Cauliflower
- Broccoli
- Mushrooms

spinach, or kale, packages of baby carrots, or pre-cut celery sticks.

- ▶ **Microwaving and steaming generally preserve more of the nutrients** in vegetables than boiling them, in which nutrients are lost to the cooking water. Roasting and grilling bring out the sweetness in many veggies; if that tempts you to eat more, it's worth sacrificing some nutrients to prolonged or high heat.
- ▶ **Beware of sauces and seasonings that can add calories,** saturated fat, and sodium to vegetables. Before buying pre-seasoned canned or frozen vegetables, check the Nutrition Facts label and/or the ingredients list to see if the product is high in sodium, calories, and/or saturated fat.
- ▶ **Look for canned vegetables labeled "reduced sodium,"** "low sodium," or "no salt added." You can further reduce the sodium content of canned vegetables by draining and rinsing them in water.

A Sampling of Super Vegetables

In the rest of this chapter, we provide more information about an array of vegetables that will help you meet your nutritional needs as you age, including tips on how to store and serve them. You may be less familiar with some items than others, such as fennel and celeriac, so consider this an invitation to experiment. Since all vegetables are good sources of a variety of valuable nutrients, select those that most appeal to your taste buds and budget.

In our list of vegetables, you'll find avocados, pumpkins, and tomatoes—foods that are technically fruits based on their botanical classification. However, since these foods are typically treated like vegetables and used in savory dishes, we're including them here. (Beans, peas, and other legumes will be covered in the chapter on protein foods.)

Artichokes

The artichoke packs a nutritional punch, though identifying the edible part is somewhat tricky for the uninformed. The tender artichoke heart is at the bottom of the vegetable. Once steamed, the cactus-like leaves can be eaten by biting down on the soft, bottom end and scraping the tender flesh into your mouth. The edible parts of the artichoke contain fiber, folate, lutein, zeaxanthin, potassium, and vitamins C and K. It is very low in calories (64 in one medium artichoke) but high in fiber, especially the soluble fiber that's been shown to improve cholesterol levels.

Select artichokes that are compact and heavy for their size, with tight leaves. To loosen the leaves of a mature artichoke, cut off the top one-third and remove the tough outer leaves by hand, then simmer in boiling water with a little lemon juice. The bases of each leaf can be eaten as well as the delicate artichoke heart. Cook only in a non-reactive pan such as stainless steel, enamel or glass, because cast-iron, copper or aluminum cookware will cause artichokes to discolor (as can carbon-steel knives).

Asparagus

Asparagus is a good source of several B vitamins, including thiamin, riboflavin, niacin, B_6, and especially folate. Low in calories, it also provides iron, potassium, and vitamin C. Asparagus contains more vitamin E than most vegetables, and it's high in dietary fiber, including a type of soluble fiber that acts as a "prebiotic," which feeds the "good" bacteria in the gut.

One downside to asparagus is that it's high in purines, which some advise gout sufferers to avoid because these compounds are thought to raise uric-acid levels. Some people also find that asparagus gives a distinctive odor to their urine, but this has no health consequences.

Select asparagus spears that are firm, with closed, deeply-colored tips. Store asparagus in the refrigerator. Thin spears aren't necessarily more young and tender; those at least a half-inch in diameter at the base are best. To extend its shelf life, place the asparagus, tips pointing up, in a container filled with about an inch of water; replace the water when it becomes cloudy.

Avocados

These days, avocados are eaten in everything from guacamole and salads to smoothies and trendy avocado toast. If you've avoided avocados because they're high in fat, think again: Of the 18.6 grams of fat in a typical avocado, only 2.9 grams are unhealthy saturated fat; the rest is heart-healthy monounsaturated fat. Research suggests that the unsaturated fat in avocados may have cardiovascular benefits. In particular, eating an avocado a day has been found to lower unhealthy LDL cholesterol.

Adding an avocado to other vegetables, such as the leafy greens in a salad, can help you absorb carotenoid compounds such as beta-carotene. One study found that topping salads with avocado boosted carotenoid absorption by three to five times.

Avocados also are being studied for joint health. They contain compounds called unsaponifiables (ASUs), and ASUs derived from avocado and soybean oils are being tested as a treatment for osteoarthritis. One study found that avocado-soybean ASUs improved symptoms of hip and knee arthritis and reduced the need for anti-inflammatory drugs. Another study reported that ASUs significantly reduced the progression of hip arthritis over a three-year period.

Avocados are good sources of several B vitamins, dietary fiber, potassium, copper, carotenoids, and vitamins C, E, and K. However, consume avocados in moderation—one cup of avocado slices contains 230 calories, a much higher calorie count than most other vegetables.

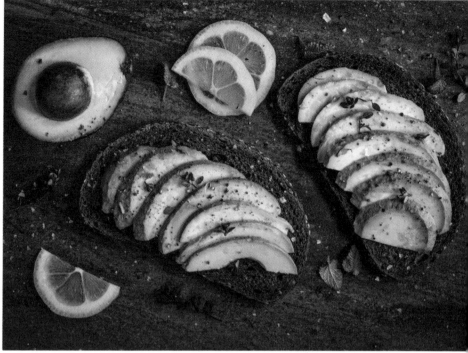

© Elena Elisseeva | Dreamstime

Avocados are high in unsaturated fat and also provide fiber and several vitamins and minerals.

Like bananas, avocados will ripen at room temperature after purchase, so choose less-ripe fruit that is firmer and less likely to be bruised. Ripe, whole avocados can be kept in the refrigerator for up to a week. Peel avocados carefully, since the greatest concentration of carotenoid compounds is in the dark-green flesh immediately under the skin.

Beets

Look for fresh beets in early summer. Nutrients are generally highest in the familiar purple-red varieties, including phytonutrients called betalains that give beets their vivid color (but which are depleted with longer cooking times). Beets also are a good source of fiber, vitamin C, potassium, folate, and iron. Although beets are high in natural sugar (hence their use in sugar production), they are low in calories.

Smaller beets are more tender and cook faster; select those that are unblemished, hard, and evenly round. Don't wash beets before storing, though you may want to trim most of the greens to reduce moisture loss. (If you also eat the greens, they are high in lutein

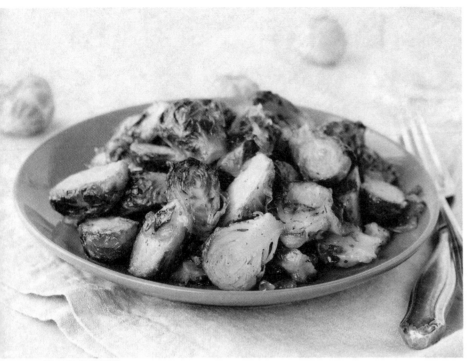
© Irenastar | Dreamstime

Roasting Brussels sprouts in the oven can bring out nutty, sweet flavors that help balance out any bitterness they may have.

help prevent stomach ulcers and inflammation by killing bacteria called *Helicobacter pylori* in the stomach. The leaves and stalks of broccoli are packed with nutrients, too, though the florets are generally the most nutrition-rich.

Research has shown that people who ate cruciferous vegetables such as broccoli were at significantly lower risk of lung cancer. Another study showed that nonsmokers who ate three or more monthly servings of raw cruciferous vegetables had a 73 percent reduced risk of bladder cancer than those who ate the fewest cruciferous foods.

Look for tightly closed, dark-green or purplish-green florets (indicating more beta-carotene and vitamin C) with tender stalks; avoid yellowing florets that are past their prime. Broccoli can be eaten raw, which retains more vitamin C, but cooking releases more carotenoids for absorption by the body. Like most of its cruciferous cousins, broccoli can be microwaved, steamed, boiled, or even roasted.

Brussels Sprouts

These suddenly trendy cruciferous veggies are high in potassium and provide thiamin, riboflavin, vitamin B6, antioxidant flavonoids, and potentially cancer-fighting phytonutrients. Pick bright-green sprouts with no cabbage-y odor; smaller sprouts are more tender and less likely to have the bitterness that makes people think they dislike Brussels sprouts. Steam Brussels sprouts, braise them in a flavorful liquid such as vegetable or chicken stock, or toss them with olive oil and roast them in the oven.

Cabbage

Another cruciferous cousin of broccoli, cabbage shares many of broccoli's nutritional benefits. All three common varieties of cabbage—red, green, and Savoy—are good sources of potentially cancer-fighting phytonutrients, along with fiber and folate. As you might guess

and zeaxanthin, which are phytonutrients that play an important role in eye health.) Peel beets only after cooking to keep their rich red color from bleeding out. When handling beets, it's smart to wear gloves and an apron, because the juice will create stubborn stains.

Like carrots, beets can be eaten raw; add shredded beets to green salads for a sweet crunch. If you're not keen on handling whole beets, you can try beet juice; this beverage has become more popular and easier to find since research found that it might help control high blood pressure.

Broccoli

The prototypical healthy veggie, broccoli is indeed a good source of nutrients, including fiber, vitamin C, calcium, folate, riboflavin, potassium, and iron. It's also high in beta-carotene and other carotenoids, such as lutein and zeaxanthin, that help protect eye health. Phytonutrients found in broccoli, such as indoles, glucosinolates, kaempferol, and isothiocyanates, are believed to have cancer-fighting properties. One phytonutrient in broccoli, sulforaphane, may from its color, red cabbage is higher in vitamin C, but Savoy cabbage contains more beta-carotene.

Select heavy, solid heads of cabbage with only a few outer wrapper leaves, which should be clean and undamaged. Hold off washing cabbage until you're ready to serve it, and don't cut with a carbon-steel knife to avoid discoloration. If cooking red cabbage, use nonreactive cookware to preserve the color.

Carrots

A single medium carrot delivers almost twice the recommended daily value of vitamin A, mostly in the form of beta-carotene. Studies have shown that beta-carotene and other carotenoids are linked with protection against conditions that can cause vision loss: For example, women who eat more carrots have lower rates of glaucoma, and animal studies have linked nutrients in carrots to a reduced risk of cataracts.

Carrots are also good sources of potassium and vitamin C, and contain calcium, zinc, and magnesium—all for just 25 calories. The fiber in carrots includes pectin, which may have cholesterol-lowering properties.

Scientists are studying phytonutrients in carrots called polyacetylenes for possible cardiovascular benefits. These compounds are thought to have anti-inflammatory properties and to keep blood cells from clumping together. Other studies are investigating these compounds' ability to inhibit the growth of cancer cells.

Look for brightly colored carrots that are smooth, firm, and relatively straight. Larger carrots are sweeter because they've had more time to develop natural sugars.

Store carrots in the coolest part of the refrigerator for up to about two weeks, wrapped in a damp paper towel and placed in an airtight container or bag. Keep carrots away from foods such as apples or pears that release ethylene gas, which will promote spoiling and bitterness. Wash carrots thoroughly before using.

Cauliflower

The plain white color of cauliflower belies its rich nutrient content. (There's also purple cauliflower, an antioxidant-rich variety that turns green when cooked, and orange cauliflower, which adds vitamin A to the equation and tastes more like winter squash.) Another mainstay of the cruciferous family of vegetables, one cup of cooked cauliflower contains 3 grams of fiber and 2 grams of protein, as well as vitamin C, folate, vitamin B_6, and potassium.

Look for cauliflower that's firm and free of bruises and blemishes, with compact florets; any leaves should be crisp and green.

Be gentle if you choose to boil cauliflower in water, as heat diminishes its vitamin C content, and its B vitamins leach into the cooking water. Roasting this vegetable brings out an earthy sweetness that may appeal to people who think they don't like cauliflower. Cooked, mashed cauliflower can be served in place of mashed potatoes or combined with them to lower the carbohydrate and calorie count. Or you can use cauliflower "rice" to make low-carb, gluten-free pizza crust.

Collard Greens

Collard greens are less familiar to Americans outside the South than other dark, leafy greens such as spinach or kale. Collards and their cousins, such as turnip and mustard greens, belong to the cruciferous-vegetable family. Among the milder of these bitter leaves, collards are a source of fiber, beta-carotene, vitamin C, folate, iron, and calcium (one of the best sources among dark leafy greens).

Shop for collards that have been kept cool, as they wilt quickly, and choose

Basic Vinaigrette

Save on calories, saturated fat, and grocery costs by whipping up your own dressing.

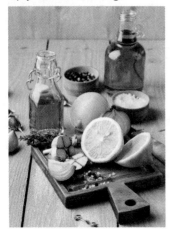

© Istetiana | Dreamstime

INGREDIENTS

2 Tbsp vinegar

½ to 1 tsp Dijon-style mustard

¼ tsp kosher salt

¼ tsp freshly ground black pepper

6 Tbsp extra-virgin olive oil (or other vegetable oil)

PREPARATION

1. Whisk together vinegar, mustard, salt, and pepper. Add the oil in a stream, whisking; continue to whisk until vinaigrette is emulsified.

2. Vary your vinaigrette by adding two tablespoons of finely chopped shallots or fresh herbs, sprinkling in some onion or garlic powder or dried herbs, or trying various types of vinegar.

smaller, tender leaves with fresh green color and no signs of discoloration. At home, wrap unwashed collards in damp paper towels and store them in the crisper. Wash thoroughly right before using and discard stems and tough leaves. Try using collards in recipes that call for cooked spinach, or add to whole grains.

Fennel

A flowering plant related to the carrot family, fennel provides vitamins A, C, and K, carotenoids (beta carotene, lutein, and zeaxanthin), fiber, and potassium. One half of a bulb has just 36 calories. While fennel is commonly used in Italian and French cooking, it is often misunderstood and neglected in the U.S. The hollow stalks are considered an herb, chopped and sautéed, then added to salads, soups, or vegetables. The part of fennel most commonly used in cooking is the cultivated bulb, called the "Florence fennel." Its inflated leaf base has a mild anise flavor with a sweeter taste. Sliced Florence fennel can be grilled, roasted, or baked.

Kale

The popularity of this leafy green member of the cruciferous family has surged in recent years. Unlike some food fads, however, kale deserves the attention: With a mere 36 calories, one cup of cooked kale delivers 5 grams of fiber and more than 100 percent of your daily vitamin A, as well as vitamins C and K, magnesium, calcium, and potassium, plus at least 45 antioxidant flavonoids. Like other cruciferous veggies, it contains glucosinolates—sulfur compounds associated with a reduced risk of cancer.

The fiber in kale is good for your digestive system, and it also benefits your arteries. Research has shown that fiber-related nutrients in kale help the liver and intestines bind cholesterol and carry it out of the body. Although raw kale can

help lower cholesterol, steam it for five minutes to get the maximum benefits from its nutrients.

Kale is typically available year-round. You'll find three common varieties:
- **Curly kale,** with ruffled, deep-green leaves and a pungent, bitter, peppery flavor.
- **Dinosaur kale,** also called Tuscan or Lacinato kale, with textured, dark blue-green leaves, and a sweeter, more delicate flavor that kale newcomers might prefer.
- **Ornamental kale,** which is edible despite its name, also is called salad savoy. Its leaves may be purple, pink, red, yellow, cream, and/or green, and it has a mild flavor and tender texture.

Select firm, deeply colored leaves with sturdy stems, free of wilting or discolored spots; smaller leaves tend to be milder in flavor. Store unwashed kale in a zip-top plastic bag in the refrigerator and use within five days, since kale's nutrient content declines rapidly.

Lettuce and Salad Greens

Generally, the darker the lettuce or other salad greens, the higher the overall nutritional content—and yet Americans eat more pale-green iceberg lettuce than kale, romaine, and spinach combined. Compared to iceberg lettuce, deeply colored greens are higher in vitamins A, C, and K, beta-carotene, the carotenoids lutein and zeaxanthin, calcium, folate, and fiber. Green and red leaf lettuces, for example, contain nearly 15 times as much vitamin A as iceberg lettuce, six times the vitamin K, almost 20 times the beta-carotene, and six times the lutein and zeaxanthin. Other popular varieties, such as romaine, Bibb, and Boston lettuce, also outshine iceberg in nutrients.

All salad greens provide vitamin C, folate, calcium, iron, and other nutrients, though amounts vary widely by type—another argument for consuming a variety. Choose the crispest salad greens you can find; in prepackaged mixes, check the sides and bottom of the container or bag for any signs of wilting, sliminess, or browning. Wrap loose salad greens in a damp paper towel and store in the refrigerator crisper, away from fruits such as apples or ripe bananas that give off ethylene gas.

Remember that even the healthiest salad can be made less healthy by slathering on dressings and other toppings high in calories and saturated fat, such as cheese and bacon. For healthier homemade dressing, try a simple recipe of whisking together one part vinegar to two parts oil. Adding a dash of mustard will help keep the oil and vinegar from separating.

Keep in mind, too, that salad greens of all sorts are prime targets for contamination with bacteria that can cause food-borne illness. Romaine lettuce, for example, has been the source of multiple headline-making outbreaks. Follow these safety tips for all varieties:

- **At the market,** place fresh greens in plastic bags to keep them separate from raw meats and poultry.
- **Refrigerate greens** at 35–40 degrees.
- **Wash hands and surfaces** before preparing salad.
- **Wash all non-prewashed greens thoroughly** under running water just before using, including produce grown conventionally or organically at home or purchased from a grocery store or farmer's market. The FDA does not recommend washing with soap or detergent or using commercial produce washes.
- **Use a salad spinner and/or blot greens** dry with paper towels.
- **If the label on packaged greens indicates that the contents are pre-washed and ready-to-eat,** the FDA says you can use the produce without further washing (which might actually expose clean greens to contaminants in the sink).

Okra

A member of the hollyhock family, this vegetable—familiar in the American South—is technically a fruit. Its gooey liquid emitted during cooking makes it a popular thickening ingredient in gumbo stew. Turned off by the goop? Cook the okra separately at high heat and then add it to the dish. This low-calorie food (12 calories for five pods) adds flavor to any meal, as well as fiber, lutein, vitamin K, and potassium.

Onions

Members of the *allium* family, onions are related to garlic, which has been extensively studied for its potential health benefits. Onions are a good source of vitamin C, potassium, and dietary fiber. They also are among the richest sources of quercetin, a phytonutrient with antioxidant and anti-inflammatory properties.

Organosulfur compounds are released by cutting or crushing the onion; in garlic, these compounds have been associated with cancer protection, improved cholesterol levels, and decreased stiffness in blood vessels. It may be that allowing onions to sit for a few minutes after cutting, prior to cooking, helps preserve these beneficial compounds, as has been demonstrated with garlic.

Research has shown that the more pungent, stronger-smelling onions, which are highest in sulfur compounds, exhibit anti-platelet activity. That might help prevent platelets from clumping together in your blood vessels, reducing the risk of atherosclerosis, stroke, and heart attack. Generally, yellow and red onions are highest in beneficial compounds, while milder (sweet or Vidalia) varieties are lowest. Those sulfur compounds, as well as quercetin, may be responsible for onions' apparent cancer-protective effects.

When selecting dry bulb onions, look for those that are firm and have little or no smell. Avoid any with cuts, bruises, or blemishes. Store unpeeled onions in a cool, dry, dark place to better preserve their antioxidant compounds. Peel your onions carefully, as the phytonutrients tend to be more highly concentrated in the outer layers.

Peas

Peas are members of the legume family (which also includes beans and lentils), so they are higher in protein than most green vegetables. Their fiber includes pectin, which may aid in combatting unhealthy cholesterol. Nutrition numbers vary by type, with green peas higher in B vitamins and zinc, while snow peas stand out for vitamin C and folate. Snow peas are lower in protein and calories than green peas.

Frozen green peas provide a go-to option for an easy vegetable suitable for side dishes, stews, casseroles, and pilafs. When buying fresh peas still in the pod, look for firm, glossy, medium-sized pods. Keep fresh peas refrigerated, as their sugars rapidly turn to starch at room temperature, and rinse thoroughly before using. Young green peas can be eaten raw along with the pods, as can snow peas and sugar snap peas.

Pumpkin

It's time to think of pumpkins beyond Halloween jack-o'-lanterns and Thanksgiving pie. Despite their high water content (90 percent), nutrient-dense pumpkins deliver a modest amount of protein and fiber, vitamins C and E, and beta-carotene—with only 49 calories in one cup of cooked pumpkin. That single cup of cooked pumpkin contains 564 milligrams of potassium—more than a banana and almost an eighth of what you need in a day. Pumpkin also provides copper, manganese, zinc, iron, selenium, and magnesium.

The pumpkin is a type of winter squash and a member of the gourd family; it works well in savory preparations,

whether it is baked, puréed in soups, or added to stews. Canned pumpkin purée is as good a choice as fresh pumpkin and far more convenient—just be sure to select 100-percent pumpkin, rather than pumpkin pie filling, which contains added sugar. If you buy a whole pumpkin, save and roast the seeds for a nutritious snack, salad topping, or granola ingredient.

Snap Beans

A favorite with gardeners, these edible-pod beans are most commonly seen as green beans or yellow wax beans; both are actually immature forms of kidney beans. Formerly known as "string beans," snap beans are now bred to grow mostly without the tough "string" down the pod's seam. Nutritionally, green beans and yellow wax beans are similar, except that the latter contain less beta-carotene. Both types are good sources of dietary fiber, potassium, vitamin C, folate, and iron.

Look for crisp, not stiff, pods of uniform size for even cooking. Thin French beans known as *haricots verts* are more tender and fast-cooking in simple sauté preparations. Trim the ends before cooking, but otherwise, keep them whole during cooking to keep nutrients from leaching out.

Spinach

Popeye was right about spinach: This leafy green nutritional powerhouse has been linked to health benefits including boosting muscle strength, reducing diabetes risk, and protecting against cataracts. Spinach is rich in carotenoids and vitamin K. It's also a good source of vitamins C and E, and B vitamins, calcium, potassium, and magnesium.

Though spinach is famously high in iron, the oxalates found in these nutritious greens interfere with the absorption of iron as well as calcium. That high oxalate content also means people at risk for the most common type of kidney stones, calcium oxalate stones, may need to limit their spinach consumption. Patients on blood-thinning medications such as warfarin should check with their physicians before changing their consumption of leafy greens, such as spinach and kale, which are high in vitamin K, which can counteract the effects of warfarin.

Buy smaller, vividly green, sweet-smelling spinach leaves with thinner stems and no signs of yellowing. Spinach, especially loose-leaf, requires rigorous rinsing to remove grit; dry in a salad spinner unless you plan to cook the spinach, which can be cooked damp. Because carotene compounds are fat-soluble, you'll get the most from your spinach when it's combined with a little heart-healthy unsaturated vegetable oil, such as olive oil in a salad; cooking also will release more of these compounds.

Summer Squash

Summer squash vary widely in appearance, color, and nutritional values, but all are gourds—relatives of melons and cucumbers. Unlike their harder-rind winter cousins, summer squash, including zucchini and crookneck or yellow squash, are picked while still immature. Their high water content leaves little room for calories, but summer squash still deliver fiber, magnesium, potassium, and vitamins A and C. The green rind of zucchini is packed with eye-protecting lutein and zeaxanthin.

Select small to medium squash that feel firm and heavy for their size and are free of nicks. Store in the refrigerator (unlike winter squash). Try grilling lightly oiled summer squash, shredding into a slaw, or adding to stir fries.

Sweet Potatoes

Sometimes mistakenly called yams, sweet potatoes are not even distantly related to the tuber that is popular in African cooking but seldom seen in the

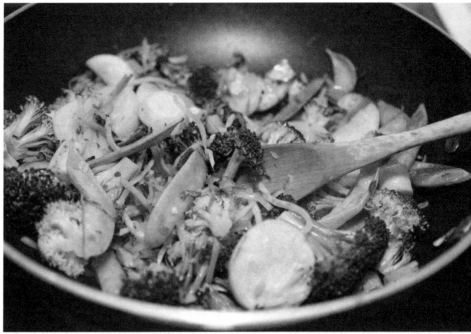

Stir-frying is a quick, healthy way to cook vegetables.

U.S. Sweet potatoes can be found in a range of colors, from pale orange to deep red and purple. Their rich, deep color indicates a high concentration of carotenoids. One cup contains enough beta-carotene to produce 769 percent of the daily value of vitamin A. That one cup also delivers 7 grams of fiber (versus 2 grams in a white potato).

A heart-healthy reason to eat sweet potatoes is their potassium content—950 milligrams in one cup. You'll also get a healthy dose of vitamins B_6 and C.

When cooking sweet potatoes, leave the skins on—that's where the majority of the phytonutrients are located. Sweet potatoes can be baked or roasted, but some data suggest that boiling them (with the skin on) results in the best conservation of nutrients and the lowest impact on blood glucose levels. While sweet potatoes are loaded with nutrients, they're starchy vegetables, which means they're higher in calories than non-starchy vegetables, so keep an eye on your portion size.

Tomatoes

Tomatoes provide more than 10 percent of your recommended daily value of

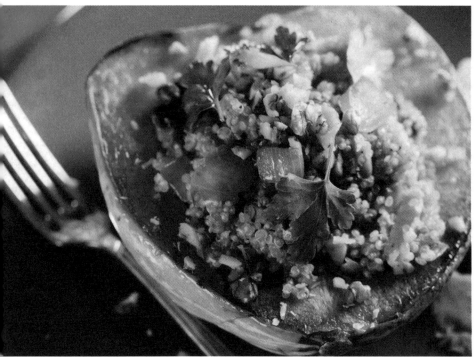

© Charlotte Lake Dreamstime

Cut winter squash in half, scoop out the seeds, bake it, and then stuff it with a mixture of quinoa, onions, mushrooms, and herbs.

better source of lycopene than raw tomatoes, because heat breaks down the cell walls in the tomatoes and releases the lycopene. Because lycopene is fat soluble, combining tomatoes with a little olive oil or other healthy fat makes it easier for your body to absorb it.

Look for smooth, plump, unblemished tomatoes with a sweet fragrance. Store fresh tomatoes in a cool, dark place such as a pantry—not in the refrigerator, where cell walls and volatile flavor compounds will break down. Tomatoes that must be refrigerated to prevent spoilage still can be used in a sauce; try putting them out on the counter for a few hours before cooking them. Canned tomatoes are a convenient option and a pantry staple; check labels to make sure your tomatoes aren't loaded with sodium.

vitamin C, vitamin K, copper, potassium, and manganese per cup, with only 30 calories. Their high potassium content may explain why tomato consumption has been associated with a reduced risk of cardiovascular disease. One cup also contains 2.2 grams of fiber—more than some breakfast cereals.

Tomatoes are an important source of phytonutrients, including the flavonols quercetin and kaempferol, which are found primarily in the skin, as well as beta-carotene and lycopene. Lycopene, the phytonutrient that gives tomatoes their rich, red color, also may contribute to cardiovascular protection. High levels of lycopene in the blood have been associated with a lower risk of stroke in men, as well as improved cholesterol and triglyceride levels. By countering the aggregation of platelets in the blood, lycopene and other tomato compounds may reduce the risk of atherosclerosis. Lycopene also may be key to tomatoes' possible anti-cancer benefits. Studies have linked high intake of lycopene with reduced risks of breast and prostate cancer.

Cooked tomatoes, including canned tomatoes and sauces, actually are a

Winter Squash

Though nutrient contents vary by species, winter squash are at least as nutritious as pumpkin and deliver more nutrients than varieties of summer squash such as zucchini. Winter squash are low in calories; for example, one cup of cooked butternut squash provides just 80 calories. They are an excellent source of carotenoids and vitamin C, and also contain B vitamins and potassium. One cup of winter squash has 6.6 grams of dietary fiber, most of it the insoluble form that promotes digestive health. The pectins and other polysaccharides in winter squash also may have anti-inflammatory and insulin-regulating properties.

All winter squash have an interior hue that falls along the spectrum of yellow to orange—a signal that, like carrots and pumpkins, they're rich in alpha- and beta-carotene, precursors to vitamin A. Some studies have rated winter squash as among the best sources of these compounds. One cup of cooked butternut squash provides nearly 23,000 IU of vitamin A—560 percent of the recommended daily value. Foods high in vitamin A may help protect against certain cancers, and vitamin A is essential to maintaining eye health. Vitamin A also supports cell growth and differentiation, playing an essential role in the maintenance of the heart, lungs, kidneys, and other organs.

Winter squash also deliver lutein, zeaxanthin, and a vitamin A precursor called beta-cryptoxanthin, which has been studied for anti-inflammatory properties and may reduce the risk of rheumatoid arthritis.

Winter squash belong to a subgroup of the *Cucurbitaceae* family of plants, the *Cucurbita* genus, whose extracts are being studied for anti-cancer properties. Compounds in *Cucurbita* foods also may inhibit an enzyme that contributes to the buildup of cholesterol.

Winter squash also serve up significant amounts of five B vitamins, including B_2, B_3, B_6, folate, and pantothenic acid. B vitamins, along with a compound called d-chiro-inositol that also is found in winter squash, are important to the body's regulation of blood sugar.

Despite their name, winter squash are at their best in autumn. Select squash that are unblemished, firm, and heavy for their size. Look for rinds that are hard (a soft rind signals a watery interior) and dull or matte, not glossy (a sign of squash picked too soon before it can sweeten). If present, the stem should be firmly attached. Along with familiar varieties, such as acorn and butternut, try other types such as buttercup, delicata, carnival, turban, hubbard, kabocha, and sweet dumpling. Try serving stringy spaghetti squash in place of pasta.

Whole winter squash can be stored in a cool, dark place for as long as six months, depending on the type. Wash the rind thoroughly in running water before using. Once cut, store in the refrigerator for up to two days, or freeze.

What About Potatoes?

You may have noticed an omission from this list—America's most popular vegetable, the potato. We consume more than 50 pounds of potatoes per person annually, more than 20 pounds more than the second-most popular veggie, tomatoes. For many Americans, potatoes—white, red, Russet, or colorful varieties such as Yukon Gold or Adirondack Blue—are a dietary staple. It's not surprising, considering that potatoes are affordable, easy to store and prepare, and filling.

However, many popular potato dishes, including loaded baked potatoes, *au gratin* potatoes, potato skins, French fries, and potato salad, often contain heaping helpings of unhealthy fat and sodium. Plain potatoes that are simply boiled, roasted, or baked have plenty of nutritional benefits; they are good sources of potassium, vitamin C, and folate. Potatoes eaten with the skin deliver fiber that can help offset the negative effects of their dietary starch. You can still enjoy potatoes; just make them one of the many vegetables you eat, and keep your portion sizes in check.

As you've seen in this chapter, there's a considerable variety of nutrient-packed vegetables available. If you've been eating the same four of five vegetables for years, now is a great time to add some new ones to your dietary pattern.

Myths vs. Facts: Nightshade Vegetables

Do you need to avoid "nightshade" vegetables if you have arthritis, as some internet buzz suggests? Vegetables from these plants in the *Solanaceae* family include peppers, tomatoes, white potatoes, and eggplants. Some say these vegetables and their botanical cousins contain compounds that aggravate arthritis pain and inflammation. It's true that these foods are related to belladonna, also called "deadly nightshade," a toxic plant infamous in history (and mystery novels) as a source of poison because of compounds called solanines. But no nightshade vegetable cultivated for human consumption has anywhere near a high enough level of solanines to cause ill effects.

Research has found no evidence that nightshades have any effect on joints or can make arthritis worse, according to the Arthritis Foundation. And nightshade vegetables are rich in nutrients, making them a worthy addition to most diets. The Arthritis Foundation even puts one group of nightshade vegetable, peppers, on its list of "Best Vegetables for Arthritis." Peppers of all types are rich in vitamin C, which may protect cells in cartilage against damage.

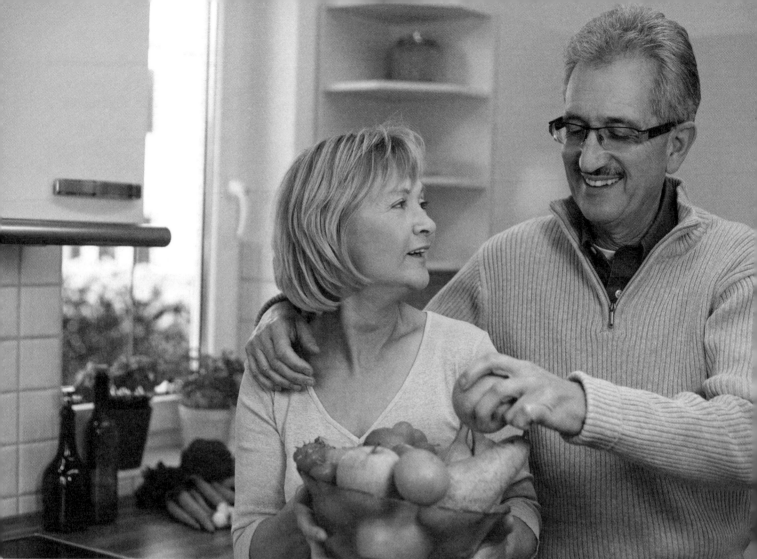

© Robert Kneschke | Dreamstime

The natural sugar in fruit can help satisfy your "sweet tooth."

5 The Power of Fruit

Including fruit in your dietary pattern may reduce your risk for heart disease and protect against some types of cancers. Fruit, along with vegetables, might also lower your risk of frailty, a condition characterized by weakness and low energy that increases your risk of falls, hospitalization, and disability, as you age. One study found that participants who ate at least five servings of fruit and vegetables a day had a 69 percent lower risk of developing frailty than those consuming only one daily serving. Participants who consumed at least three daily servings of fruit had a 52 percent lower risk of frailty than those who consumed none.

Eating fruit can help you pass up less healthy choices, too, which is why they make smart snacks and desserts. One study found that women of normal weight were more likely to keep fresh fruit out on the kitchen counter, while women who were overweight or obese were more likely to have boxed cereals, cookies, chips, or soft drinks sitting on their counters.

Don't Fear Fruit's Sugar

Because fruits taste so sweet, some people think they can't possibly be as good for you as vegetables. People with type 2 diabetes, in particular, often believe they should avoid fruit because it contains naturally occurring sugar. The American Diabetes Association, however, advises: "Fruits are loaded with vitamins, minerals, and fiber just like vegetables. Fruit contains carbohydrate, so you need to count it as part of your meal plan. Having a piece of fresh fruit or fruit salad for dessert is a great way to satisfy your sweet tooth and get the extra nutrition you're looking for."

In fact, consuming certain fruits—including blueberries, grapes, and apples—at least three times a week has been linked to a lower risk of diabetes. The fiber in whole fruits helps decrease the rate at which glucose (sugar) is released into the bloodstream.

Fruit also is associated with a lower risk of obesity. One study found that participants with dietary patterns characterized by higher intakes of fruit were 12 percent less likely to be obese than those with lower fruit intakes. (On the other hand, people who had a diet higher in sugary soft drinks and chocolate were about 9 percent more likely to be obese.) The researchers commented, "Natural sugars, such as in fruits, and added sugars, such as in sugar-sweetened drinks, are chemically similar, but research suggests they have opposite effects on our health. This is because the combination of other nutrients that make up the food (and your overall diet) is very important. Fruits should be encouraged as they are an important source of many beneficial nutrients, such as potassium and fiber."

A Good Source of Antioxidants

Another reason to consume fruit that's much touted in commercials—especially for juice products—is the miraculous-sounding power of antioxidants. But before you buy "super" beverages or supplements packed with antioxidants, realize that these nutrients are just another reason to eat an overall healthy diet. And it's better to eat whole fruits with their fiber intact than to drink juices, especially juices with added sugars.

Antioxidants include such familiar nutrients as vitamins C and E,

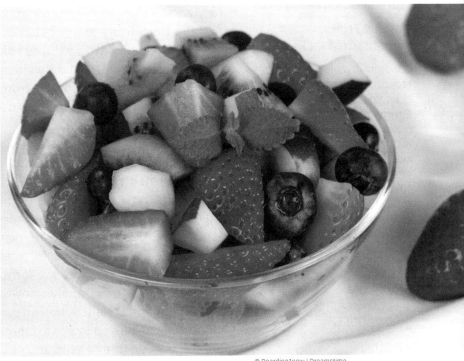

© Boarding1now | Dreamstime

All fruits are good sources of antioxidants.

carotenoids such as beta-carotene, and the mineral selenium, as well as many different phytonutrients, notably polyphenols. Antioxidants neutralize substances called "free radicals," some of which are natural byproducts of the body's use of oxygen. Other sources of free radicals include cigarette smoke, pollution, radiation, and some pesticides and cleaning products. Antioxidants reduce the "oxidative stress" that is caused by an excess of free radicals and the associated damage to DNA believed to contribute to diseases.

Antioxidant Benefits. Some observational studies have reported that antioxidants might reduce the risk of cardiovascular disease and some cancers. Laboratory tests show that antioxidants may slow or possibly prevent cancer development, according to the National Cancer Institute.

Numerous studies suggest that eating fruit and other healthy foods rich in antioxidants is associated with health benefits. Higher dietary intake of vitamins C and E and selenium has been linked to a sharply lower risk of pancreatic cancer, for instance. A diet rich in antioxidants, especially from fruits and vegetables, has been associated with a reduced risk of stroke. And, in a 2018 study, women with higher antioxidant intake from foods such as fruits and vegetables were at lower risk of developing diabetes.

Don't Count on Supplements. Researchers have learned that the benefits of antioxidants now seem to be more complex than simply fighting free radicals. That complexity may explain disappointing—or worse—results in tests of the same compounds in pill form. One controversial meta-analysis even reported that antioxidant supplements were associated with an increased mortality risk. A large trial of supplemental vitamin E and selenium was halted over concerns that the treatments were doing more harm than good. Smokers should avoid extra beta-carotene, which can increase lung cancer risk.

The most recent negative findings include a sweeping review of supplementation studies in the June 2018 *Journal of the American College of Cardiology*. No benefit in cardiovascular disease outcomes and all-cause mortality was seen for extra vitamin C, beta-carotene, or selenium, among other supplements.

The best advice seems to be to consume plenty of foods high in antioxidants, which may have more beneficial functions than fighting free radicals, and to skip the supplements. Oranges and other citrus fruits, strawberries, and kiwifruit are among the best sources of vitamin C. You can get plenty of beta-carotene and other carotenoids in orange-colored fruits such as cantaloupe, peaches, and apricots. Berries of all types, as well as grapes, are excellent sources of polyphenols. In general, eating fruit with the skin, in which polyphenols are most concentrated, is the best way to get the most antioxidants from fruits such as apples, pears, and plums.

Getting Enough Fruit

How much fruit should you consume? According to the USDA, women over age 50 should aim for one-and-a-half cups of fruits daily, and men over 50 should try for two cups. People who are physically active may need even more. In general, one cup of fruit, a half-cup of dried fruit, or an 8-ounce glass of 100-percent fruit juice counts as "one cup" of fruit; one small apple, a large orange or peach, a medium pear, or one large banana also is equivalent to "one cup."

In Tufts' MyPlate for Older Adults, fruits play a prominent role for several reasons. Fruits are sources of many essential nutrients, including potassium, dietary fiber, vitamin C, and folate, and they are rich in phytonutrients, the beneficial plant compounds discussed in the previous chapter. Fruits contain no cholesterol and minimal or no saturated fat or sodium, and they are low in calories. Two cups of apple slices, for example, contain about the same number of calories as five Hershey's kisses.

Increasing Your Consumption

It's easy to increase your intake of healthy fruits. Keep a bowl of whole fruit on the table or kitchen counter. Pre-cut packages of fruit, such as melon or pineapple chunks, make handy snacks. Dried fruits are easy to pack in lunches or for munching on the go.

As with vegetables, frozen fruit is at least as nutritious as fresh, since it's picked at the peak of ripeness, and freezing locks in nutrients that otherwise deteriorate over time. If you buy canned fruits, make sure to choose those packed in water or 100-percent juice with no added sugar.

The USDA's MyPlate offers these tips for including more fruits in your diet from breakfast to bedtime:

- ▶ **At breakfast,** top your cereal with fruit, add blueberries to pancakes, or mix fresh fruit with plain yogurt.

- **Make a fruit smoothie** for breakfast or a snack by blending fat-free or low-fat milk or yogurt with fresh or frozen fruit. Try bananas, peaches, strawberries, or other berries. (Note that, unlike "juicing," puréeing fruits in a blender preserves the dietary fiber.)
- **For lunch,** pack fruits protected by peels (bananas, oranges, tangerines) for safe transport, or take containers of single-serving fruits (choose products that contain no added sugar).
- **For fresh fruit salads,** mix apples, melon, grapes, and berries with acidic fruits like grapefruit or pineapple, or add lemon juice to prevent browning.
- **At dinner,** add fresh or dried fruits to green salads. Try meat dishes that incorporate fruit, such as chicken with apricots or fish with mango salsa, or add chunks of pineapple or peaches to kabobs.
- **For dessert,** have baked apples, pears, or a fruit salad.

Fruit Favorites

In the rest of this chapter, we highlight the nutritional and health benefits of a variety of fruits. Of course, these are just examples—your supermarket's produce section is packed with other good choices. For the best value and nutrient content, buy whatever fruit is in season.

Apples

This fruit is famously said to "keep the doctor away"—and apples actually are beneficial to your health. One meta-analysis concluded that eating one or more apples a day was linked with lower risks of many types of cancer compared to consuming less than one apple a day. Similarly, in a large U.S. population study, the number of servings of apples and pears eaten was correlated with a reduced risk for lung cancer.

Apples are high in phenolic acids and flavonoid compounds—phytonutrients that may protect against cell and DNA damage. In the laboratory, these compounds have been found to inhibit growth of cancer cells, decrease lipid oxidation, and lower cholesterol.

Experts recommend washing apples well so you can consume the peel as well as the flesh. Apple peels contain the majority of phytonutrients compared to the flesh, and peels add an extra boost of fiber. While storage doesn't affect the levels of most phytonutrients, processing does. If whole fruit isn't an option, cloudy, unsweetened apple cider has significantly higher amounts of phytonutrients than clear apple juice. (Don't risk unpasteurized cider, however, which may harbor dangerous microorganisms.)

Select firm apples that are free of soft spots or bruises. Apples keep best in the crisper of a refrigerator with a damp cheesecloth added for moisture. Apples do lose some nutrients over months of storage, but they retain enough to remain a healthy choice.

Apples produce ethylene gas, which can cause other fruits and vegetables to become overripe, so keep apples separated from other produce whenever possible.

Blueberries

The MIND diet, mentioned in chapter 2, specifically advocates consuming more berries, and blueberries are among the most-studied for brain benefits. For example, researchers analyzed data on strawberry and blueberry consumption among 16,010 women over age 70 and found that women with the highest intake of berries experienced slower mental decline than women who ate the fewest berries.

Polyphenol compounds in blueberries also may help normalize blood pressure, according one study of postmenopausal women with early-stage hypertension. Women who consumed freeze-dried blueberry powder—equivalent to eating a cup of berries a day—averaged

NEW FINDING

Blueberries vs. Blood Pressure

A study reports that eating 200 grams of blueberries every day for a month can lead to an improvement in blood vessel function and a decrease in systolic blood pressure in healthy people. That's more than a cup a day of blueberries, but scientists say the results show the power of the anthocyanin pigments that give the berries their blue hue. Researchers from King's College London studied 40 healthy volunteers who were randomly given either a drink containing blueberries or a matched control drink daily. Effects on blood vessel function were seen two hours after consumption of the blueberry drinks. Over the course of a month, blood pressure was reduced by 5 mmHg—similar to what is commonly seen in studies using blood pressure-lowering medication. The researchers noted, "If the changes we saw in blood vessel function after eating blueberries every day could be sustained for a person's whole life, it could reduce their risk of developing cardiovascular disease by up to 20 percent."

The Journals of Gerontology: Series A, Feb. 16, 2019

7 mmHg lower systolic blood pressure (the top number in a blood-pressure reading) than a control group after eight weeks.

Other clinical trials are testing blueberries' possible benefits for vision, gout protection, arterial function, blood sugar, and more. Research has suggested that blueberries may have a positive effect on cardiovascular health by improving cholesterol levels.

Blueberries are rich in anthocyanins, the phytonutrients that give them their distinctive color, as well as quercetin, kaempferol, ellagic acid, and resveratrol, and they provide vitamins C and K, manganese, and dietary fiber.

Choose firm, uniformly colored berries, and don't be concerned if you see a whitish bloom on the berries—that's a natural coating that protects their skins. Keep fresh berries in a covered container in the refrigerator, and don't wash them until just before eating them.

Frozen is fine for blueberries: Research has shown that frozen blueberries retain most of their anthocyanin content. Cooking at temperatures above 350 degrees Fahrenheit damages these polyphenols, however, so keep that in mind if you add blueberries to muffin, pancake, or quick-bread batters.

Cranberries

Don't limit your cranberry consumption to Thanksgiving. The polyphenol compounds in cranberries include high levels of anthocyanins, which contribute to the berries' bright red color. Processing, such as in making cranberry juice, does cause some loss of these and other phytochemicals. High heat also can damage compounds in cranberries.

In terms of health benefits, cranberries are probably best known for their effects against urinary tract infections (UTIs). Several studies and two meta-analyses have supported the effectiveness of this long-standing folk remedy, but other studies have failed to find a link between cranberry intake and reduced UTI recurrence.

Another promising, if lesser-known, area of research into cranberries' possible health benefits relates to cardiovascular health. Studies have shown cranberries might protect the heart and blood vessels by improving cholesterol, combating oxidative stress, decreasing inflammation and inflammatory compounds, and reducing arterial stiffness. Cranberries also seem to improve the function of the lining of blood vessels and increasing levels of nitric oxide, which dilates blood vessels.

Grapes

Botanically, grapes are in the berry family, and they are rich in anthocyanins (especially red and purple grapes), much like similarly-colored berries, so scientists have theorized that grapes and grape juice may have brain benefits similar to those associated with berries. Some research suggests that grapes and berries may have beneficial effects on the ways that neurons in the brain communicate. By boosting the brain's signaling functions, the anthocyanins and other phytochemicals in these fruits may prevent damaging inflammation in the brain and have a protective effect on cognition and motor control. Tufts researchers have previously reported that Concord grape juice reversed brain aging in rats.

Other studies have linked health benefits with moderate consumption of red wine, but if you'd rather not tipple, you can probably get similar health advantages from plain grape juice. Red grape juice (made from red and/or purple grapes) contains the same phytonutrients as red wine, which help improve blood vessel health and protect against high blood pressure.

Grapes contain resveratrol, a compound that has been associated with boosting memory and preventing platelets from clumping together. As with all fruit juices, though, be wary of the high sugar content in grape juice. Although fruits contain natural sugar, fruit juices lack the fiber found in whole fruits that helps slow the rate at which glucose (sugar) enters your bloodstream.

Guava

We've included this less-familiar fruit because it's a nutritional powerhouse. Guavas are the fruits of an evergreen shrub or small tree. Guavas grown in Florida are at their peak from August through October and in February and March.

One cup of guava pieces provides more than six times the daily value of vitamin C, with the highest concentrations found in the flesh just under the rind. Guava is also the tropical fruit with the highest potassium content, with nearly 20 percent of the daily value per cup—more than is found in a comparable amount of the famously potassium-rich banana. Potassium can help control blood pressure and regulate your heart rate, and consuming more potassium has been linked with a lower stroke risk.

The pink color of guavas is a clue that they are one of the few fruits high in lycopene, an antioxidant carotenoid that also gives tomatoes their red color. By weight, guavas contain nearly twice the lycopene of tomatoes. Lycopene has been associated with lower stroke risk, reduced markers of inflammation, and improved cholesterol and triglyceride levels, and may help protect against prostate cancer.

Kiwifruit

Like the people of New Zealand, known as "kiwis," the kiwifruit is named for the flightless bird native to that country. Originally grown in China and known as "Chinese gooseberries," this fruit came to New Zealand with missionaries

in the early 20th century and was renamed upon introduction to the U.S. in the 1960s. Kiwifruit from New Zealand can be found on supermarket shelves from June through October; fruit from California is available from November through May.

The bright green flesh, speckled with tiny black seeds, contains more vitamin C per cup than an orange. Kiwifruit has been studied for its antioxidant properties, which research has indicated may help ease asthma symptoms such as wheezing and shortness of breath in children. In one study, volunteers who ate two or three kiwifruit a day for four weeks showed an 18 percent improvement in platelet aggregation response, an indicator of a reduced risk for blood clots, and a 15 percent reduction in triglyceride levels.

Consume kiwifruit soon after cutting and add to fruit salads just before serving, as enzymes released by slicing cause it and nearby fruits to soften. Kiwifruit contain oxalate, a substance that can combine with calcium and produce kidney stones or gallstones. If you've had either of these stones, ask your doctor what type they were; if they were calcium oxalate stones, limiting your intake of oxalate may help prevent more stones from forming.

Mangos

Mangos are among the world's most widely consumed fruits, and they are available year-round due to the many varieties that are grown. The golden-yellow flesh reveals that mangos are high in beta-carotene, which is a precursor to vitamin A. Diets high in beta-carotene have been associated with a lower risk of certain cancers. Mangos also are a source of zeaxanthin,

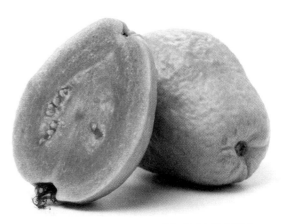

Depending on the variety, guavas may have pink or white flesh, and they may be round, oval, or pear-shaped.

a carotenoid compound associated with eye health.

Unripe mangos will continue to ripen on the counter; lightly squeeze the fruits to test ripeness rather than relying on color. To serve, slice close and parallel to the seed on either side to make two halves. With the skin side down, cut a checkerboard pattern in the flesh of each half, and then run a spoon or knife between the flesh and the skin to pop off the pieces.

Some people have an allergy to a chemical compound called urushiol that is found in the skins of mangos, so make sure no skin remains on the flesh. As an added precaution, rinse the mango flesh before eating it, and wash your hands thoroughly after handling a mango and/or wear gloves when peeling it. (Incidentally, urushiol is the compound in poison ivy and poison oak that causes allergic reactions; if you're allergic to these plants, you may be more likely to be allergic to mangos.)

Oranges

Practically synonymous with vitamin C, oranges deliver about 130 percent of the recommended daily value per fruit. Vitamin C is vital for the body's production of collagen, a key connective protein found in bones, teeth, and cartilage. Vitamin C is also an antioxidant that may prevent cell damage. One orange also provides 12.5 percent of the recommended daily value of dietary fiber—most of which is lost if the orange is squeezed into juice.

But it's not all about the vitamin C. Oranges contain a wealth of other, lesser-known phytonutrients, including:

- **Beta-cryptoxanthin,** a carotenoid that helps give oranges their distinctive color, has been associated with a reduced risk of lung cancer.
- **Limonoids,** which have been studied for cholesterol-lowering benefits and anticancer properties.
- **Polymethoxylated flavones,** found in the orange's peel, which significantly lower unhealthy cholesterol levels in laboratory animals.
- **Zeaxanthin,** which may help reduce your risk of rheumatoid arthritis (RA).

Buy oranges with smoothly textured skin that are firm and heavy for their size, which indicates a higher juice content. Smaller fruit with thinner skins are typically juicier. Fully ripened oranges are highest in nutrients, including carotenoids and flavonoids. Don't worry about non-uniform peel color (perfect-looking oranges may get that way from Citrus Red #2 dye), but do avoid mold or soft spots.

Store oranges loose rather than in a plastic bag. Oranges last about two weeks with little loss of nutrients whether they are kept in the refrigerator or at room temperature.

Papaya

Native to Central America but now grown throughout the tropics, papayas are at their peak from early summer into fall. Most supermarket papayas come from Hawaii, but you also may see the much larger, less intensely flavored Mexican variety. Partially ripe fruit will continue to ripen on the counter (you can speed the process by placing near an apple or a banana); ripe papayas will keep a day or two in the refrigerator.

Almost as rich in vitamin A as mangos, papayas also are a source of lycopene. One study found that men who drank green tea and also consumed tropical fruits, including papayas and guavas, were at lower risk of prostate cancer.

Papayas contain an enzyme called papain that helps digest proteins and can be used to tenderize meat; papain also may have anti-inflammatory effects. Concentrations are highest in green papayas.

Peaches

Peaches are one of the many fruits with a high water content, which translates into a modest calorie count—there are only 39 calories in a medium-sized peach. But peaches still pack plenty of nutrients: One medium peach contains two grams of fiber—mostly in the form of soluble fiber, shown to improve cholesterol levels. Eating a peach gives you more than 10 percent of your recommended daily intake of vitamins A and C, plus modest amounts of B vitamins, vitamin E, vitamin K, potassium, and minerals. Antioxidant phytonutrients in peaches include lutein, zeaxanthin, and beta-cryptoxanthin.

Peaches have not been studied as extensively as have some other fruits. However, lab tests have shown that polyphenol compounds in peaches (as well as plums) selectively killed breast-cancer cells, leaving healthy cells unharmed. Other researchers have found that peach extracts slowed the growth of aggressive breast-cancer cells in mice.

Shop for peaches that are richly colored, and free from blemishes or bruises. Ripe fruits yield to gentle pressure with the whole hand and have a sweet smell. Unlike some fruits, peaches will continue to ripen after picking; keep underripe peaches at room temperature and store them in a paper bag to hasten ripening. Ripe peaches can be stored in the refrigerator but are best brought to room temperature before eating to maximize their flavor. Wash peaches in cold water just before using. You'll obtain the most nutrients by eating the whole peach, including the skin.

Strawberries

Strawberries are packed with healthy phytonutrients as well as essential vitamins and minerals, and they're the world's most popular berry variety. Studies have linked strawberry anthocyanins to improved blood vessel function and lower blood pressure. The phytonutrients in strawberries also may reduce levels of C-reactive protein (CRP), a marker of inflammation that's associated with several chronic health conditions, including cardiovascular disease.

Surprisingly, one cup of strawberries (about eight whole berries) contains more vitamin C than a medium orange—about 140 percent of the recommended daily value. A cup of strawberries also delivers more than a quarter of your daily manganese, an essential nutrient that must be obtained from your diet. Manganese helps your body process cholesterol, carbohydrates, and protein, and it plays an important role in bone formation.

Strawberries have a very short shelf life; their nutritional content drops sharply after just a few days, and they deteriorate rapidly. Buy medium-sized, fully ripe fruit; underripe strawberries aren't as nutritious and won't ripen further after picking. Store unwashed, unhulled strawberries in a cold, humid part of the refrigerator, preferably in a sealed container, and wash them thoroughly before eating.

If your meal plans change and you're not going to eat the strawberries within a few days of buying them, wash them thoroughly, cut in halves or quarters, place them in a tightly sealed plastic bag, and store them in the freezer.

It's fine to eat whichever fruits are your favorites, and all of the examples listed here are nutrient-rich choices. Remember, though, that the greater variety of fruits (and other foods) you eat, the wider diversity of nutrients you get. Other healthy fruits include bananas, cherries, grapefruit, melons, blackberries, plums, apricots, and pineapple.

Peaches provide several vitamins and minerals, as well as antioxidants.

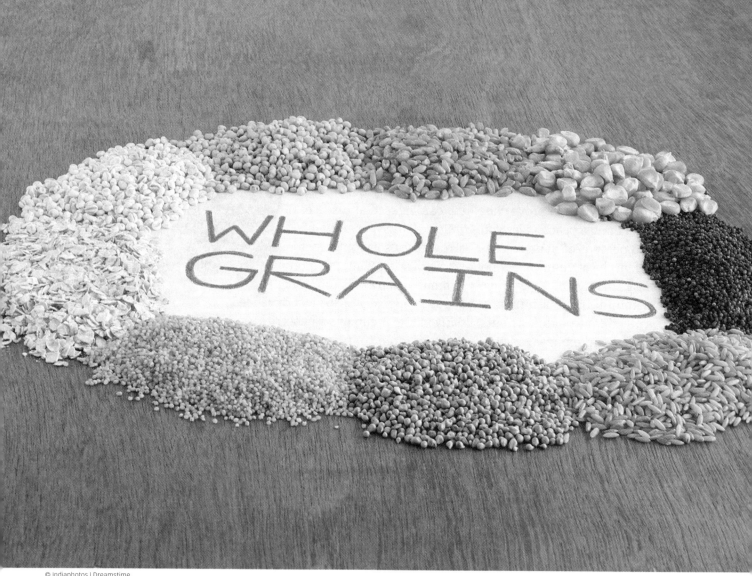

Incorporate a variety of whole grains into your diet to boost your fiber and nutrient intake.

6 Healthy Fiber and Whole Grains

You may think of fiber as something only old people need enough of to combat constipation, but research continues to show that dietary fiber—along with whole grains, which contain fiber and other nutrients—does much more for your body than just keep you regular, regardless of your age.

In one study, for example, participants with the highest intake of dietary fiber had an almost 80 percent greater likelihood of "successful aging," defined as reaching old age free of chronic disease, disability, cognitive impairment, symptoms of depression, and respiratory symptoms. In the study, the group of participants with the highest total fiber intake averaged 37 grams per day, while those in the group with the lowest intake averaged only 18 grams daily.

You probably aren't getting 37 grams of daily fiber—and it's likely you may not even be consuming the recommended minimum amounts. The daily recommended fiber intake is 38 grams for men ages 18 to 50 and 25 grams for women ages 18 to 50. Calorie needs decrease as you get older, as we've noted, and so does the recommendation for fiber; for men and women over age 50, it drops to 30 grams per day and 21 grams per day, respectively. The "% Daily Value" (% DV) for fiber shown on Nutrition Facts labels has been based on a recommendation of 25 grams of fiber per day, but that number will be increased to 28 grams as nutrition labels are updated. The change reflects research demonstrating the cardiovascular benefits of increased fiber intake.

Despite these recommendations and the research, most Americans fall short of even the lowest fiber targets. The average American eats only 10 to 15 grams of fiber per day, and fewer than 5 percent of all Americans get enough fiber in their daily diets.

Not Just Cereal

You get fiber from various plant sources in your diet, including vegetables, fruits, nuts, seeds, and grains. Fiber from grains is known as "cereal fiber," a term that applies to the fiber in foods such as brown rice, millet, barley, and bulgur wheat, as well as to your morning breakfast cereal. Higher cereal fiber intake is associated with a lower risk of cardiovascular disease and a decreased risk of dying after surviving a first heart attack.

Although this chapter focuses on fiber and other nutrients from healthy grains, you shouldn't overlook other sources of fiber. The fiber naturally found in fruits and vegetables, for example, is why you should skip the "juicing" trend—which leaves that fiber behind—and consume whole fruits and veggies. Beans and other legumes, which we'll cover in the chapter on protein, are especially rich in fiber; one cup of cooked black beans, for example, has 15 grams of fiber. Even nuts and seeds can contribute significantly to your daily fiber intake: An ounce of almonds (about 23 nuts) contains 3.5 grams of fiber.

Greater intake of dietary fiber aids in regulation of blood glucose levels, which in turn contributes to better heart health and a reduced risk of diabetes (diabetes is a risk factor for heart disease). Research also has shown that consuming soluble fiber (the type that absorbs water) modestly reduces levels of LDL ("bad") cholesterol in your blood.

Fiber also may help reduce your risk of cancer, particularly in the digestive system. Many, but not all, studies have reported an association between greater fiber intake and lower incidence of colorectal cancers.

Consuming fiber can make you feel full more quickly and help the feeling of fullness last longer. As a result, you may eat fewer total calories, which reduces your risk of obesity and heart disease.

What About Added Fiber?

Some food manufacturers have added fiber to their products to entice health-conscious shoppers to buy their brands. But are these added fibers as good for you as naturally occurring fiber from grains, nuts, and produce?

"Many consumers are not aware that some of these added fibers may not have the same physiological health benefits as fibers found naturally in plant foods," says Nicola McKeown, PhD, a scientist with Tufts' Nutritional Epidemiology program and an associate professor at the Friedman School. For example, research studies have suggested that the added fibers psyllium and beta-glucan are effective at reducing cholesterol, but inulin (sometimes called chicory root) appears to have no effect on cholesterol levels (although it may have some benefit as a prebiotic).

Unlike natural fibers found in foods, added fibers (also called isolated fibers) must be included on ingredient lists. Isolated fibers commonly added to processed foods include pectin, guar gum, psyllium, cellulose, and inulin (often sourced from chicory root).

The FDA recently reviewed the scientific literature to determine which added or isolated fibers are associated with health benefits including lower blood glucose and cholesterol levels, lower blood pressure, regularity, increased absorption of minerals in the intestinal tract, and calorie control. The FDA review identified these added fibers as providing these benefits: beta-glucan, psyllium husk, cellulose, guar gum, pectin, locust bean gum, and hydroxypropyl-methylcellulose. Further, the FDA announced it intends to propose that eight other non-digestible carbohydrates, including inulin, be added to the definition of dietary fiber.

Make Your Grains Whole

Fiber is only part of the reason to prefer whole grains, however. Switching your breakfast cereal, upgrading your sandwich bread, and giving the grains on your dinner plate a makeover could help protect your heart. Whole grains have been associated with reduced risk of cardiovascular disease, better cholesterol levels, and lower blood pressure. People who eat more whole grains are also at lower risk of cancer, respiratory disease, infectious diseases, diabetes, and early death.

What makes a grain food "whole"? Whole grains contain all parts of the entire original grain kernel—the bran, germ, and endosperm. Contrast that with refined grains that have been milled, a process that removes the bran and germ to give the flour made from the grain a finer texture and a longer shelf life. During this process, significant amounts of nutrients are lost, including fiber, iron, and many B vitamins.

Many products made with refined grains are enriched, however, meaning that certain B vitamins (thiamin, riboflavin, niacin, folic acid) and iron—but not fiber—are added after the grain has been milled. Although whole grains are the healthiest choice, if you are going to buy refined-grain products, check the ingredient list to make sure that the word "enriched" is included in the grain name (for example, "enriched wheat flour"). Some grain products are made from mixtures of whole grains and refined grains. Not all whole grains are particularly high in fiber—cooked brown rice has only 2 grams per one-half cup, for example. But whole grains are higher in all sorts of nutrients, and even those relatively low in fiber exceed the amount in processed, refined alternatives: Cooked white rice contains a meager 0.6 grams of fiber per one-half cup.

How Much Do You Need?

The 2015-2020 *Dietary Guidelines for Americans (DGA)* recommends making at least half your grains whole grains. For most people, the total recommended daily intake is six servings of grains, so three or more servings of your daily grains should be whole. Grains include the grains themselves, such as oats or barley, as well as foods in which grains are an ingredient, such as bread or pasta.

Servings (called "ounce equivalents" in the *DGA*) are described in kitchen measures. Examples of one serving of whole grains include one slice of bread, one-half cup of cooked oatmeal, pasta, quinoa, bulgur wheat, or wild rice, and three cups of air-popped popcorn.

Benefits of Whole Grains

If you need convincing to switch from familiar white sandwich bread to whole wheat, or from white rice to brown rice, barley, or farro, consider recent research

---

What Grains Are Whole?

According to the Whole Grains Council, the grains below, when consumed in a form including the bran, germ, and endosperm, are examples of generally accepted whole-grain foods and flours:

• Amaranth	• Farro/emmer	• Quinoa	• Triticale
• Barley	• Freekeh	• Rice (brown)	• Wheat
• Buckwheat	• Kamut	• Rye	• Wheat berries
• Bulgur	• Kañiwa	• Sorghum	• Wild rice
• Corn	• Millet	• Spelt	
• Einkorn	• Oats	• Teff	

Many of these grains make a heart-healthy substitute for white rice. You can serve alongside stir fries, pack into burritos, or turn grains into pilafs or risottos. Just make sure to leave plenty of cooking time, as with brown rice, since most whole grains take longer.

findings. Like cereal fiber in general, whole grains can help improve unhealthy cholesterol levels. In one analysis of 24 randomized controlled trials, study participants who consumed whole grains had lower "bad" LDL cholesterol and total cholesterol levels overall than participants who did not eat whole grains, and they also tended to have lower triglyceride levels. Whole-grain oats had the greatest beneficial effects. The longer the participants consumed whole grains, the greater were their improvements in LDL and total cholesterol. Other studies have linked consumption of several specific varieties of whole grains, including oats, barley, sorghum, and amaranth, to healthier cholesterol levels.

Even if you're already taking a statin medication to improve your cholesterol levels, Tufts research has shown that you can reap additional benefits from consuming more whole grains. In one study, statin users who consumed more than 16 grams a day of whole grains had healthier cholesterol levels than statin patients who ate fewer whole grains.

In other research, whole grains were found to help protect against aortic stiffness, even among people who are overweight or obese. Aortic stiffness is a thickening or hardening of the body's main artery and it is a significant predictor of heart disease, heart failure, and stroke. The study, focused on obese men, reported that of all food choices, greater intake of whole grains was the only factor significantly associated with less aortic stiffness.

Another study reported a strong association between greater whole-grain consumption and a lower risk of chronic diseases. Consuming five to six servings daily of whole grains (was associated with a lower risk of death from cancer, respiratory disease, diabetes, and even infectious diseases. People whose diets were rich in whole grains were also at a lower risk of coronary heart disease,

cardiovascular disease, and stroke, as well as deaths from those causes. Even a modest intake of one or two servings a day of whole grains was associated with health benefits.

Getting Your Whole Grains

To start consuming more whole grains, look for ways to swap them for less healthy choices rather than adding them to the grains you're already eating. The goal isn't to eat more food, but to eat healthier food that contains more nutrients.

The recommendation is to eat 48 grams or more of whole grains daily. According to the Whole Grains Council, each of these food servings will provide you with about 16 grams of whole grains:

- One-third cup of cooked whole-wheat pasta
- One-third cup of cooked brown rice, bulgur, barley, or other cooked grain
- One slice of whole-grain bread
- Half of a whole-grain English muffin
- 4 Triscuit crackers
- Two-thirds cup of Cheerios
- One-third cup of Wheat Chex
- Two-fifths cup of cooked oatmeal

Whole Grains Labeling

To make sure you're buying whole grains, look for a Whole Grain Stamp from the Whole Grains Council. The ingredients list is another reliable source of information; look for phrases such as "100% whole [name of grain]." (Just because a food product is made with whole grains doesn't guarantee that it is healthy, however; continue reading to see if the product contains added sugar or salt.)

All of these ingredients indicate that a product contains whole grains:

- Whole grain [name of grain]
- Whole wheat
- Whole [name of grain]
- Stoneground whole [grain]
- Brown rice

Whole Grain Stamps

The Whole Grains Council has created three stamps to help consumers identify foods that contain whole grains. Some breads and other grain products carry these stamps on their packaging. The "100% Whole Grain" stamp indicates that the product contains all whole grains and/or whole-grain flours, the "50%+ Whole Grain" stamp means that more than half of the grains in the product are whole grains, and the "Whole Grain" stamp indicates that the product contains at least some whole grains. Each stamp also provides the minimum number of grams of whole grains found in one serving of the product. If there's no stamp, that doesn't mean that the food does not contain whole grains; food manufacturers are allowed to use Whole Grains Stamps on food packaging only if they're a member of the Whole Grains Council.

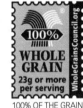

100% OF THE GRAIN
IS WHOLE GRAIN

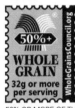

50% OR MORE OF THE
GRAIN IS WHOLE GRAIN

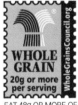

EAT 48g OR MORE OF
WHOLE GRAINS DAILY

Fiber in Whole Grains

GRAINS	FIBER* (GRAMS)
Barley (hulled)	8
Farro (not pearled)	7
Bulgur wheat	6
Cornmeal	5
Cracked wheat	4
Steel-cut oats	4
Popcorn (air-popped, 3 cups)	4
Quinoa	3
Brown rice	2

*Per ¼ cup dry (½- to ¾-cup cooked) except as noted

- Oats, oatmeal (including steel-cut, old-fashioned, quick-cooking, and instant oatmeal)
  - Buckwheat (even if it isn't preceded by the word "whole")

Ingredients that indicate only a "maybe" include wheat, wheat flour, semolina, durum wheat, and organic flour. Other "maybe" terms are "stone-ground" (without "whole"), and the ubiquitous "multi-grain." Ingredients that never mean whole grains include enriched flour and degerminated corn meal. If you see wheat germ or oat bran, it typically indicates that supplemental fiber was added to the product.

Cooking Whole Grains

What befuddles many novices about whole grains is cooking time. Because whole grains include the tougher outer layers of the grain, they sometimes take more time (and often more liquid) to cook. However, several grains, including quinoa, buckwheat, and bulgur wheat cook in 20 minutes or less.

If you can cook regular white rice, you can master whole grains, as the basic techniques are the same: Combine a dry grain in a pan with water or broth, bring to a boil, and simmer until the liquid is absorbed. (Pastas made from whole grains are cooked just like regular spaghetti, with extra water drained away before serving.)

You can get a little fancy by toasting whole grains in a few teaspoons of olive oil before adding the cooking liquid. Or make a simple pilaf by browning finely chopped onions and other vegetables in a little oil, adding the grain, and then stirring in broth.

Some planning can reduce the cooking time, too: Just soak the grains in water for a few hours before mealtime. When it's time to prepare dinner, top off the pan with more water or drain the water and add broth, and then bring to a boil and simmer until the grains are tender.

Some of the hardiest grains require an overnight soak prior to cooking.

Another time-saving strategy is to cook a big batch of whole grains and store the leftovers for later meals. Cooked grains will keep three or four days in the refrigerator and up to four months in the freezer. Add a little water and reheat in the microwave, or use in soups or cold salads.

Pre-cooked whole grains, such as 90-second brown rice, make side dishes as simple as moving a package from your pantry to the microwave.

Smart Substitutions

Start your day with whole grains by building breakfast around them. Having a bowl of hot oatmeal means you've already got one serving of whole grains—but consider other whole-grain options for variety. For example, you can make porridge with amaranth, barley, teff, or millet, or create breakfast bowls with quinoa, cornmeal (not degerminated), or wheat berries.

Not all hot cereals are whole-grain choices, however. While all versions of oatmeal, from instant to steel-cut, are whole grain, some popular hot cereals, such as the original Cream of Wheat (farina) and the original Cream of Rice, are not whole grain. (Cream of Wheat has, however, introduced a special whole-wheat version.)

Even when you're buying a whole grain such as oatmeal, the way it's processed can make a difference. Steel-cut oats are the best choice for supplying your body with the slow, steady stream of glucose that supports good health.

Steer clear of flavored oatmeal products, which usually are high in added sugar. Instead, buy plain cereals and add your own finishing touches, such as fruit or nuts. Even if you add a touch of sugar, honey, or maple syrup, you'll end up with less added sugar than in the packaged, sweetened varieties that contain as much as 12 grams, or three teaspoons, of sugar per serving. Spices such as cinnamon and nutmeg also can help enhance the flavor.

Ready-to-eat breakfast cereals can deliver whole-grain nutrition, too, but you'll need to be a label detective. Look at the ingredients for the whole-grain terms discussed earlier in this chapter, and check to make sure the first item in the ingredients list is a whole grain. (Hint: If the first ingredient is sugar, it's not a healthy choice.) Don't assume "multi-grain" ready-to-eat cereals are whole-grain choices.

Include whole grains in your lunchtime sandwiches simply by choosing whole-wheat rather than white bread. If you're concerned about calories, you can find ultra-slim whole-wheat options with as little as 45 calories per slice, or sandwich "thins" that provide 100 calories total. Or, skip the bread and choose whole-grain flatbreads or tortillas. Even burgers can be made healthier by switching to whole-wheat buns.

A Variety of Whole Grains

The world of whole grains ranges from such familiar foods as wheat, oats, and corn to more exotic varieties like quinoa and farro. Here are some examples of whole grains that will help provide you with the fiber and nutrients you need for healthy aging.

Corn and Popcorn

Americans eat a lot of corn, a versatile food that can be a grain, a vegetable, a source of cooking oil, and the main ingredient in a common sweetener.

"With respect to meal planning, sweet corn falls under the vegetable category," says Tufts expert Nicola McKeown, PhD, who is also a scientific advisor to the Whole Grains Council. "The dried, ground corn we eat in foods such as corn bread, grits, and polenta falls under the grain category. Make sure cornmeal, corn flour,

grits, corn tortillas, and polenta packages have 'whole corn' or 'whole grain corn' listed as an ingredient; degerminated corn is not a whole grain."

When corn is dried and milled, it is considered a grain. Whole-grain cornmeal or corn flour is higher in vitamin A and carotenoids and slightly lower in dietary fiber than other whole grains, such as whole wheat or whole rye.

Popcorn also is considered a grain. "Air-popped popcorn is an excellent whole-grain snack that provides dietary fiber," Dr. McKeown notes. Adding butter and salt makes popcorn decidedly less healthy, so try eating it plain, or use just a teaspoon of butter (or a spritz of butter-flavored cooking spray) and a sprinkle of salt if you can't resist.

Although corn is a "starchy" vegetable that is high in carbohydrates and natural sugars (9 grams per cup), it releases sugar into the bloodstream steadily rather than causing a spike in blood sugar due to its fiber content. The American Diabetes Association includes it as a "best choice" among starchy vegetables as well as whole grains.

Cooked corn is a good source of fiber, potassium, and niacin. One cup of corn contains almost 5 grams of protein—more than a comparable serving of broccoli, for example. Yellow corn contains lutein and zeaxanthin, two carotenoid antioxidants that are important to eye health.

Quinoa

Once virtually unknown in the U.S., quinoa can now be found in a variety of colors (white, red, black) and forms (grains, flakes, cereals, pasta) in most large supermarkets. Though it's touted as a "super grain," this ancient Incan staple isn't technically a grain at all; it's the seed of a plant related to spinach, beets, and chard.

What makes quinoa such a nutritional standout? Quinoa ranks highest among all grains in potassium (159 milligrams

Quinoa Basics

Keep uncooked quinoa in a dry, airtight container. Storing quinoa in the refrigerator rather than the pantry prolongs its shelf life up to six months.

Quinoa seeds are protected from pests and the elements by a bitter, soapy coating called saponin. By the time it reaches grocery stores, most quinoa has had the saponin removed—but it's still a good idea to give the grains a quick rinse and rub them together with your hands to remove any lingering traces.

Quinoa's tiny grains are ready to eat in just 15 minutes. Place one part quinoa and two parts water in a saucepan, bring to a boil, cover, reduce the heat to low, and simmer until the grains turn translucent and their little white "tails"—the crunchy germ—pop out. Fluff with a fork and serve. For a nuttier flavor, lightly toast quinoa in a dry pan for five minutes before cooking. Raw quinoa expands three to four times in volume when cooked.

Quinoa is a versatile grain that can be used in a variety of dishes, much like rice. Serve warm quinoa as a side dish instead of potatoes, chill it and mix with vegetables, beans, and herbs for a cool summer salad, or stir it into vegetable soups or chili to boost fiber and protein content.

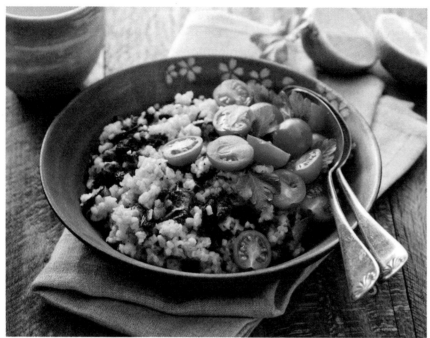
© Elena Veselova | Dreamstime

Bulgur wheat is very versatile; add your choice of vegetables and seasonings and serve as a hot side dish or a cool summer salad.

in one-half cup), a mineral associated with reducing high blood pressure. It's high in iron and most B vitamins and is a good source of zinc, copper, magnesium, and manganese.

Quinoa is also one of only a handful of plant foods that supplies all the amino acids in adequate amounts necessary for a "complete" protein. Quinoa has an unusually high ratio of protein to carbohydrates, since its protein-rich germ makes up about 60 percent of the grain. A half-cup of cooked quinoa packs more than 4 grams of protein. It's also gluten-free, making quinoa a nutritious option for people with celiac disease.

Wheat and Wheat Varieties

The average American eats more than 100 pounds of wheat flour per year. Much of that is refined, however, meaning we're missing out on nutrients: Whole-wheat flour contains 13 grams of fiber, 16 grams of protein, and 436 milligrams of potassium per cup, plus 41 percent of your daily magnesium. Compare that to 3 grams of fiber, 13 grams of protein, 134 milligrams of potassium, and 7 percent of daily magnesium in a cup of refined, all-purpose flour.

In addition to switching to whole-wheat flour and breads, you can explore many varieties and forms of wheat, including bulgur, farro, Kamut (khorasan), einkorn, spelt, and wheat berries. (Despite its name, buckwheat is not a type of wheat; instead, it's a seed that does not contain gluten.) Each of these grains has a slightly different texture and taste; here is a brief description of a few members of the wheat family.

Bulgur, or bulgur wheat, consists of whole-wheat kernels that have been steamed, dried, and cracked but have retained all of their nutrients. In America, bulgur is perhaps best known as the main ingredient in the popular Middle Eastern dish tabbouleh, which usually contains tomatoes, lemon juice, olive oil, and fresh herbs and is served as a cold salad. Since the grain kernels have been cracked, bulgur cooks more quickly than some other whole grains, in 10 to 15 minutes.

Farro is often referred to as an "ancient grain," since historical records indicate that it has been around for thousands of years. Farro and other ancient grains such as spelt, millet, and amaranth have been "rediscovered" in recent years by chefs and others in the food industry who have embraced the trend of integrating ancient grains into modern culinary styles.

When buying farro, avoid products that are "pearled" or "semi-pearled"; these terms indicate that some or all of the outer bran has been removed from the grain. (This is also the case with "pearled" barley.)

Wheat berries are wheat kernels from which the outer husks have been removed. They have a chewy texture and a slightly nutty flavor. Wheat berries, which take about an hour to cook, can be served hot as an accompaniment to chicken, fish, or beans, or cooled and combined with vegetables, fruits, nuts, and/or seeds for a filling summer dish. Like other varieties of wheat, wheat berries are a good source of plant protein, so you can use them as a base upon which to build a meatless meal.

The Gluten-Free Craze

These days, it seems everybody is "going gluten-free." For people with celiac disease, avoiding gluten—a protein found in wheat, rye, and barley—is a medical necessity. In celiac disease patients, gluten triggers an immune reaction that damages the small intestine and decreases nutrient absorption. It is believed that about 3 million Americans have celiac disease. However, many people who have celiac disease are undiagnosed; diagnosis requires a blood test and, sometimes, further testing to confirm inflammation in the small intestine.

Robert M. Russell, MD, emeritus professor at Tufts' Friedman School, advises, "If you are having a problem with intermittent abdominal bloating and pain, unintentional weight loss, or chronic diarrhea, you should consult your doctor.... It is not prudent, however, to attempt to diagnose yourself by cutting out gluten-containing foods to see if you feel better. This can actually make celiac disease more difficult to clinically diagnose."

Many people have adopted a gluten-free diet because they believe avoiding gluten will help them feel healthier or lose weight, even though they don't have celiac disease. However, in terms of nutrition, gluten-free grains are no healthier than grains that contain gluten.

Nutrient Shortfalls

Should you go gluten free? Pamela Cureton, RD, LDN, a research dietitian at the Center for Celiac Research, says, "There is no evidence that gluten is harmful in healthy people without a gluten-related disease." Moreover, gluten-free diets can come up short on nutrients. A report from the American Dietetic Association cautioned that gluten-free products averaged lower amounts of B vitamins, calcium, iron, zinc, magnesium, and dietary fiber than products that contain gluten.

Many food manufacturers would like you to believe that "gluten-free" is synonymous with "healthy," but there are plenty of gluten-free junk foods, including chips, snack foods, and sweets, that are packed with calories, sugar, and/or sodium. Going to a gluten-free bakery and indulging in cupcakes, cookies, or pies is no healthier than getting similar products at a conventional bakery.

If you don't have celiac disease, there's no scientifically valid reason to deprive yourself of the nutrition you'll get from consuming moderate amounts of wheat, barley, and rye, especially in their whole-grain forms.

Wheat Is Not Unhealthy

Similarly, you may have heard that eating wheat contributes to abdominal fat (so-called "wheat belly") or even hurts your brain ("wheat brain"). But there's no cause for concern: There is nothing inherently unhealthy in wheat.

"It is true that Americans overconsume *refined* wheat products—energy-dense, nutrient-poor foods that are high in sugar and fat—so wheat is often a 'co-passenger,'" says Dr. McKeown. "Yes, cutting out these refined foods will lead to weight loss. However, the trouble lies in the message that wheat is the culprit. There is a lack of scientific evidence to support the claims that eating wheat is an independent risk factor for greater abdominal adiposity or weight gain." What is actually important, she says, is learning how to identify whole-grain options that replace refined grains in your diet.

Research by Dr. McKeown and colleagues has shown that substituting whole grains for refined grains is associated with less—not more—belly fat. If you're trying to lose weight, limiting processed foods that contain refined wheat flour, along with sugar and saturated fat, also can be helpful.

As for the notion that eating wheat may increase your risk of Alzheimer's disease, that simply doesn't stand up to scientific scrutiny. After all, grains, including wheat, are key foods in both the DASH dietary plan and the Mediterranean-style diet, and research has linked both regimens to a *lower* risk of dementia.

A Note on the Glycemic Index

Another concept in popular diets, the glycemic index (GI), has more solid science behind it. However, recent research has cast doubt on how reliable or useful this measurement might be as a tool for weight loss and avoiding or managing diabetes.

The GI is simply a score of how rapidly carbohydrates in specific foods boost blood glucose (sugar). But Tufts researchers have previously found that GI measurements vary widely, making them unreliable dietary guides. And a new Tufts study reveals that what you eat with high-carb foods also can skew blood-glucose effects.

Scientists looked at how blood glucose and insulin levels were affected by adding foods with different amounts of carbohydrate, protein, fat, or fiber to a standardized portion of white bread, which has a high GI because it's low in fiber and digested quickly. They found that the blood-glucose impact of a high-carbohydrate food was blunted when eaten with a high-protein food. That's likely because protein slows stomach emptying, so glucose from carbohydrates enters the bloodstream more slowly. The researchers commented, "This suggests that glycemic index values, which by definition do not account for other foods eaten at the same time, shouldn't be used in isolation to modify your food choices."

Instead of chasing the latest food fads, make an effort to consistently choose whole-grain, high-fiber foods and substitute them in place of processed, low-fiber products. You don't need a fad-diet book to eat better as you age—just a keen eye for nutrition labels.

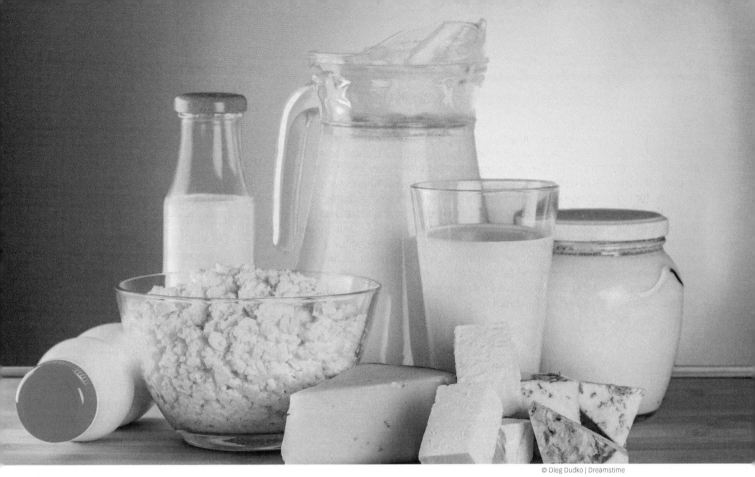

© Oleg Dudko | Dreamstime

7 Dairy Do's and Don'ts

The advertising slogan "Milk—it does a body good" may have been put on the shelf, but the fact remains that milk and other dairy products deliver significant nutritional benefits. Tufts' MyPlate for Older Adults includes dairy products such as milk and yogurt, because these are excellent sources of nutrients you may not be getting enough of as you age. These nutrients include calcium and (in fortified dairy products) vitamin D for healthy bones, protein to keep you strong, and potassium for heart and vascular health. Foods in the dairy group also contain phosphorus, vitamin A, riboflavin, vitamin B_{12}, zinc, choline, magnesium, and selenium.

Dairy Benefits

Research has linked dairy consumption with many health benefits. Consumption of dairy products is linked to improved bone health and may reduce the risk of osteoporosis. Research continues to show that dietary sources of calcium are the most effective and safest way to obtain this mineral that is essential to bone health.

Consuming dairy products also is associated with a reduced risk of cardiovascular disease and type 2 diabetes, and with lower blood pressure in adults.

Low-fat dairy consumption has been linked to a reduced risk of frailty—defined as exhaustion, weakness, low physical activity, slow walking speed, and unintentional weight loss. In one study, participants age 60 and older who consumed seven or more servings per week of low-fat milk and yogurt had a 48 percent lower incidence of frailty than those who consumed less than one serving per week. Consuming whole milk or full-fat yogurt or cheese, however, was not linked to lower frailty risk.

Consuming milk, primarily fat-free or low-fat milk, also has been associated with reduced progression of

Low-fat or fat-free dairy products contain the same amount of calcium, protein, and other nutrients as full-fat products but with fewer calories and less saturated fat.

Dairy Linked to Lower Heart Disease and Mortality Risk

The large, multinational PURE study of 136,000 individuals (ages 35-70) across 21 countries reported that consuming milk, yogurt, and cheese was associated with reduced risks of cardiovascular disease and death. Compared to no dairy intake, consuming more than two daily servings of dairy was linked to a 16 percent lower risk of death or a major cardiovascular event. Results were the same for full- and low-fat dairy products, and consumption of saturated fat from dairy sources did not significantly increase risk. Even having more than one but less than two daily servings of milk or yogurt was associated with lower risk. The PURE study has been controversial, and an accompanying editorial cautioned that the findings are "not the ultimate seal of approval for recommending whole-fat dairy over its low-fat or skimmed counterparts. Readers should be cautious and should treat this study only as yet another piece of evidence (albeit a large one) in the literature."

The Lancet, November 24, 2018

Dairy: What Counts as a Cup

Serving sizes of dairy foods that are equivalent to one cup include:

- 1 cup (8 ounces) of milk, yogurt, or milk alternative
- 1½ ounces of natural cheese
- 2 ounces of processed cheese
- 2 cups of cottage cheese
- ½ cup of ricotta cheese
- ⅓ cup of shredded cheese

osteoarthritis. Again, no benefit was seen for other dairy products, and cheese consumption was linked to increased arthritis progression.

Changing Tastes

Despite these benefits and the efforts of dairy marketers, Americans' consumption of milk has declined. According to a U.S. Department of Agriculture (USDA) report, however, dairy consumption has dropped 40 percent since 1970, and each younger generation is consuming less milk than the one before. Non-dairy beverages made from soy, rice, almonds, coconuts, and cashews have made significant gains in the market share. At the same time, the popularity of yogurt, especially Greek yogurt, has boomed.

The *2015-2020 Dietary Guidelines for Americans* made reference to these changing tastes and trends, advising, "Healthy eating patterns include fat-free and low-fat (1%) dairy, including milk, yogurt, cheese, or fortified soy beverages (commonly known as 'soymilk')." The guidelines recommend that adult men and women of any age should aim for three cups of dairy or the equivalent per day. Here are some strategies to help you get those three cups:

▶ **Use fat-free or low-fat milk** instead of water to make oatmeal and hot cereals.

▶ **Make smoothies** by combining yogurt with fruit and ice in a blender.
▶ **Include fat-free or low-fat milk** or calcium-fortified milk alternatives as a beverage at meals.
▶ **Use yogurt as the base** for dips for fruits or vegetables.
▶ **For dessert,** make pudding with fat-free or low-fat milk, or top cut-up fruit with yogurt.

To minimize your risk of food-borne illness, avoid raw (unpasteurized) milk or any products made from raw milk.

Possible Downsides to Dairy

Not everything in milk and other dairy foods is necessarily good for you, however. Whole milk and products made from whole milk, including butter, cream, cheeses, and yogurts, are contributors to dietary saturated fat. That's why the USDA's MyPlate advises, "Choose fat-free or low-fat milk, yogurt, and cheese. If you choose milk or yogurt that is not fat-free, or cheese that is not low-fat, the fat in the product counts against your limit for calories from saturated fats."

But these recommendations are controversial, as some research has challenged the choice of reduced-fat dairy products. One study, for example, followed the development of type 2 diabetes among more than 3,000 adults over two decades. Those with the highest initial level of dairy fat in their bloodstream actually had about a 50 percent lower risk of diabetes than those with the lowest amounts.

Another surprising study reported that middle-aged men who consumed high-fat milk, butter, and cream were significantly less likely to become obese over a period of 12 years than their peers who avoided whole-milk dairy products. A meta-analysis of 16 observational studies similarly associated whole-fat dairy intake with a lower risk of obesity.

One possible explanation for these counterintuitive results is that the fat in dairy products makes you feel "full" and less likely to eat other, less-healthy foods such as starchy, salty snacks. Dariush Mozaffarian, MD, DrPH, dean of Tufts' Friedman School and a co-author of the dairy and diabetes study, says there's evidence that "when people consume more low-fat dairy, they eat more carbohydrates" as a way of compensating.

As the science sorts itself out, Dr. Mozaffarian says, advice "should be neutral about dairy fat, until we learn more."

Calories and Added Sugar Cautions

It is true that reduced-fat dairy products contain fewer calories than full-fat versions of the same products, simply because fat is a concentrated source of calories. One cup of skim milk has only 83 calories, compared to 149 calories in one cup of whole milk. Fortunately, when the fat is removed from milk, the nutrients remain intact; skim, 1%, and 2% milk all have as much calcium and protein as whole milk. Also make sure your dairy choices have been fortified with vitamin D—not all yogurts, for example, are good sources of vitamin D.

Some yogurt products also contain high amounts of added sugars, making them nutritionally more like a dessert than a healthy choice. Check the Nutrition Facts panel: A 6-ounce container of plain, low-fat yogurt contains about 12 grams of natural sugars (from the lactose in milk), and the same serving size of plain, low-fat Greek yogurt contains about 6 grams. Numbers much higher than those indicate added sweeteners, which you can identify by checking the ingredients list.

Easy on the Cheese

Even as Americans have been drinking less milk, we've been eating more cheese than ever before. Recent USDA reports put U.S. cheese consumption at the highest levels since the agency began tracking it in 1975. Americans eat cheese on burgers, pizza, and sandwiches, in dips and sauces, and with crackers as snacks.

Cheese is a good source of protein (6 to 8 grams per serving in most varieties) and calcium (most varieties provide between 200 and 450 milligrams per serving). However, one serving of most varieties of regular, full-fat cheese contains 7 or 8 grams of saturated fat: That's about 50 percent of your total recommended daily saturated fat—just 16 grams for a 2,000-calorie-per-day diet, according to the American Heart Association.

If you eat cheese often, keep your portion sizes in check and opt for reduced- or low-fat cheeses, which contain 25 to 70 percent less saturated fat than full-fat versions. Cheese also may make it harder to keep your sodium intake under control; for example, one ounce of cheddar cheese contains about 175 milligrams of sodium.

Healthy News on Yogurt

We've already mentioned yogurt, which is a prime example of good-for-you dairy. Tufts researchers have found that eating yogurt—even just a couple of times a week—might substantially reduce your

Saturated Fat in Cheese	
CHEESE	**SATURATED FAT (GRAMS)***
Bleu (blue)	8
Brie	7
Cheddar	8
Cheddar, low-fat	4
Feta	6
Gouda	7
Mozzarella, whole milk	7
Mozzarella, part skim	4
Muenster	8
Muenster, low-fat	5
Parmesan	7
Provolone	7
Provolone, reduced-fat	5
Swiss	8
Swiss, low-fat	4
Cheese, American, pasteurized process	6
Cheese, American, pasteurized process, 2% milk	3

*Per 1½-ounce serving
Source: USDA National Nutrient Database and manufacturer's websites

NEW FINDING

Mediterranean Diet Plus Dairy Is Beneficial

One drawback of the Mediterranean diet is that it may not meet recommendations for calcium and dairy intake. But a randomized, controlled, crossover study reports that adding dairy to the diet still results in cardiovascular benefits. The study assigned 41 participants, age 45 and older, to a Mediterranean diet plus three to four daily servings of dairy for eight weeks; they also followed a low-fat control diet for eight weeks. One serving of dairy was defined as a cup of low-fat milk, 200 grams (about 7 ounces) of low-fat yogurt, and no more than one portion of cheese; butter and cream didn't count. Following the Mediterranean diet plus dairy led to improvements in markers of cardiovascular risk. Compared to the control diet, both systolic and diastolic blood pressure dropped (1.6 mmHg and 1mm Hg). "Good" HDL cholesterol levels increased significantly, and the ratio of total to HDL cholesterol improved. Triglycerides also dropped. If you're trying to eat more like a Mediterranean but worry that you're not getting enough calcium for bone health, add some low-fat milk or yogurt to your daily diet.

American Journal of Clinical Nutrition, December 2018

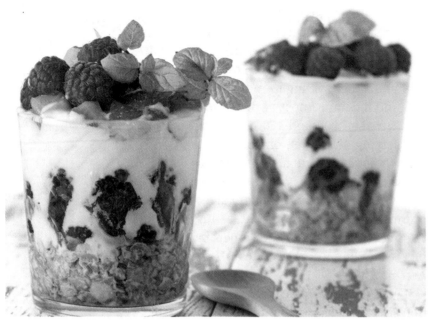

© Nazar Bignazik | Dreamstime

Make a yogurt parfait by layering fresh berries and whole-grain cereal or granola with plain yogurt.

risk of developing high blood pressure. People who consumed at least 2 percent of their daily calories from yogurt were 31 percent less likely to develop hypertension over a 14-year period than people who consumed less yogurt. (In a 2,000-calorie daily diet, you'd need to eat only two cups of plain yogurt per week to add up to 2 percent of total calories.)

Other studies have reported that yogurt eaters have lower levels of circulating triglycerides and blood glucose. People who consume more than three servings of yogurt per week appear to be better able to manage their weight. Yogurt also has been linked with better bone health: One study found that eating more than four servings of yogurt a week was associated with higher bone mineral density and fewer hip fractures.

Yogurt is a nutrient-dense food, which may be why yogurt eaters are less likely to be deficient in vitamins B_2 and B_{12}, calcium, magnesium, and zinc. The acidity of yogurt also makes it easier for the body to absorb some nutrients, including calcium, zinc, and magnesium. And depending on what type of yogurt you choose, a 6-ounce portion provides between 8 and 17 grams of protein (Greek yogurt is highest).

Good-for-You Bacteria

Yogurt is simply milk that has been fermented using cultures of "friendly" bacteria. This makes yogurt a "probiotic"—a fermented food containing healthful bacteria that promote the growth of similarly good-for-you bacteria in the body, especially in the gastrointestinal tract. For a refrigerated product to be labeled as yogurt under U.S. Food and Drug Administration (FDA) regulations, it must be cultured using two strains of bacteria, *Lactobacillus bulgaricus* and *Streptococcus thermophilus*, although other bacteria may be included. (This criterion does not apply to frozen yogurt or "yogurt products," such as candies or dips.) Although all yogurts begin with live bacteria, they don't all end with them: Some manufacturers heat-treat their yogurt after fermentation to prolong shelf life or alter the taste, which kills the beneficial bacteria.

To make sure you're getting yogurt's probiotic benefits, look for the "Live & Active Cultures" seal from the National Yogurt Association, which identifies products that meet a certain threshold of the two primary yogurt bacteria. Even if your yogurt's label doesn't have this logo, it may contain live cultures; check the ingredients for names of bacteria (for example, *Bifidobacterium lactis, Lactobacillus casei, and Lactobacillus acidophilus*), or look for a blurb on the label that mentions live and/or active cultures.

As a probiotic, yogurt may affect the community of more than a trillion microbes called the "microbiome" or "microbiota" that inhabit your intestines. Mounting evidence suggests that the bacteria in your gut affect far more than your intestinal health. The composition of the microbiota is believed to play a role in immune response, susceptibility to certain cancers or infectious diseases, and perhaps even allergies, obesity, and diabetes.

Some studies suggest that consuming yogurt with live bacteria supports digestive health and may ease symptoms of irritable bowel syndrome, as well as helping treat and prevent conditions associated with antibiotic use, such as diarrhea and yeast infections. Another bonus is that the bacteria in yogurt break down the sugars (lactose) in the milk, making yogurt a food that can be more easily digested by those with lactose intolerance.

Greek and Icelandic Options

In 2008, the thicker style of yogurt called "Greek" yogurt accounted for only 4 percent of U.S. yogurt sales; today, that market share is above 50 percent. Despite the name, Greek yogurt usually isn't imported; the thicker style is simply what is most common in many Mediterranean countries. Greek yogurt starts out the same as regular yogurt, by adding bacteria to milk. To make it "Greek," the yogurt is then strained to remove much of the liquid whey, leaving behind a thicker product.

The FDA does not regulate the term "Greek yogurt," so check ingredients carefully to make sure you're buying the real thing. Some so-called "Greek" yogurt is actually regular yogurt that's thickened with pectin, corn starch, and/or gelatin, rather than being strained.

The extra straining alters Greek yogurt's nutritional profile in some ways. Since it's more concentrated, Greek yogurt has more protein and saturated fat per ounce, but fewer carbohydrates and sugars, since some of these are removed with the whey. Some calcium is lost along with the whey, too. Amounts vary—check the Nutrition Facts label—but a typical plain, nonfat yogurt supplies about 300 milligrams of calcium, versus only 150 milligrams for plain, nonfat Greek yogurt.

Like other yogurt, Greek yogurt is made from milk that has not been fortified with vitamin D, so it's not automatically a source of this vitamin. Some brands, however, add vitamin D to all of their yogurt products.

Greek yogurt isn't just for snacking and spooning. Its thicker, creamy texture makes it a perfect substitute for mayonnaise, cream, or sour cream. Its acidic quality means it can stand in for buttermilk, and it works well in dips, as well as boosting the degree of leavening (how much the dough rises) in quick-bread or muffin recipes.

You also may see Icelandic-style yogurt in your supermarket's dairy section. Technically, this is an Icelandic cheese called "skyr," made from skim milk and bacterial cultures and then strained. Its nutritional properties are almost identical to Greek yogurt, meaning it's a good source of protein and calcium. Skyr is made with different bacterial cultures than Greek yogurts, and it is even thicker and tastes a little sweeter than Greek yogurt.

There are also Australian-style yogurts that are sweetened with honey and flavored with fruit (except for the plain varieties). This style of yogurt reportedly is based on yogurt made in Australia (although two companies that make it are in Colorado and California); it is not strained but thickened in other ways, and it is said to be creamier than Greek yogurt.

Plant-Based Milk Alternatives

The market for plant-based alternatives to dairy products continues to grow as lactose intolerance, dairy allergy, veganism, environmental concerns, and other factors lead Americans to look for alternatives to dairy. Where do these beverages fit into a healthy dietary pattern?

To understand the nutrient profiles of plant-based beverages, it helps to know how they are made. The raw materials (nuts, grains, legumes, or

Choosing Your Yogurt

Shopping for yogurt isn't as simple as it used to be. Choices these days include fat-free, 0-percent, low-fat, light, 2-percent, whole-milk, and cream-top; Greek-style, custard, Icelandic, organic, or Australian; and cow's milk, goat's milk, or no dairy milk at all. How do you choose the best option? "Your best bet is to choose yogurt in its most simple, plain form," advises Alicia Romano, a clinical dietitian at Tufts' Frances Stern Nutrition Center. "Start with plain yogurt and then control what you add."

While fat content has traditionally been the focus of yogurt labeling and advertising, Romano says what consumers should really be paying attention to is added sugar. She notes, "A lot of fat-free products tend to contain more sugar to boost the flavor."

Non-dairy yogurts, often made from soy, coconut, or almond milks, may have more added sweeteners and stabilizers to mimic the taste and consistency of dairy yogurt.

Watch out for marketing that distracts from nutritional content. For example, organic yogurts are just as likely as conventional ones to be high in added sugar.

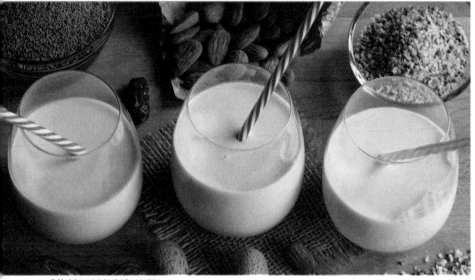

© Madeleinesteinbach | Dreamstime

Several varieties of plant-based "milks" are now available.

seeds) are soaked in water and ground (or ground and then soaked). The resulting slurry is strained to remove solids, and then flavorings, sweeteners, thickening agents (such as locust bean gum, carrageenan, or xanthan gum), stabilizers, and desired nutrients such as calcium can be added. The products then undergo heat treatment that kills any microorganisms.

The nutritional properties of these beverages depend on the plant source, processing, and fortification. A plant source like hemp, for example, may provide omega-3 and omega-6 fatty acids, and soymilk may contain soy isoflavones, which have been purported to be associated with a range of health benefits. Most milk substitutes are fortified with calcium and vitamins (such as vitamins A and D) to make them more similar to cow's milk.

Nutritional Trade-Offs

If milk substitutes are being used to replace cow's milk in the diet, it's important to be aware that they are not nutritionally equivalent. Only soy has a protein level approaching that of dairy, for example, with 7 grams of protein per one-cup serving, just slightly less than whole milk's 7.7 grams per one-cup serving. However, not all non-dairy choices are equally high in protein. Dairy also has more phosphorus, potassium, and vitamin B_{12}.

You should also be aware that drinking almond milk is not equivalent to eating almonds, for example. While whole plant foods are rich in beneficial compounds such as micronutrients and fiber, many of these (particularly fiber) are lost when they are processed into drinks.

When choosing plant-based beverages, be aware that some contain significant amounts of added sweeteners. Calories vary among plant-based milks, with sweetened, flavored varieties significantly higher, so check the Nutrition Facts label.

If you have food allergies, choose your plant-based beverages carefully: Many people who are allergic to dairy protein also are allergic to soy, and people with nut allergies should avoid nut-based beverages. Also, high levels of inorganic arsenic have been found in many rice crops, and one study found levels of this contaminant above the standard limits for drinking water in all 19 rice milks tested.

On the plus side, if you're concerned about saturated fat and don't like skim, 1%, or 2% milk, plant alternatives might be worth a try. Some varieties of plain, unsweetened plant milks contain only 30 calories per cup. The most popular alternative, soymilk, has only 0.5 grams of saturated fat per cup.

Close-up on Soymilk

As the best-selling dairy alternative, soymilk—a milky liquid produced from pressing ground, cooked soybeans—has been most thoroughly scrutinized for its health pros and cons. The most common concern about soymilk centers around phytonutrients called isoflavones that are found in soybeans.

Isoflavones are a form of plant estrogens. Although they are not identical to the estrogen hormone produced in human bodies, at one time, consuming plant estrogens was linked with the possibility of a higher cancer risk. However, recent research has largely dispelled these concerns. The American Cancer Society advises, "Moderate consumption of soy foods appears safe for both breast cancer survivors and the general population, and may even lower breast cancer risk."

Moreover, soy protein may have a protective effect against heart disease, and studies have linked it to lower LDL ("bad") and higher HDL ("good") cholesterol levels.

On the other hand, soymilk is much higher than cow's milk in phytic acid, which may reduce absorption of some minerals. Patients taking medication such as levothyroxine (Synthroid) for an underactive thyroid (hypothyroidism) should be aware that soy protein may inhibit the absorption of these drugs. If you take any medication, let your doctor or pharmacist know if you're making the switch to soy so they can check for potential interactions.

Almond Milk: A Nutty Alternative
Another popular alternative milk comes from almonds. Almond milk is low in saturated fat but contains heart-healthy mono- and polyunsaturated fats, much like the nuts from which it is made. When fortified, almond milk contains roughly as much vitamin D and vitamin A as dairy milk, and, typically, about two-thirds the amount of calcium; it has no vitamin B_{12}, however, and less phosphorus and potassium than dairy.

Almond milk is the lowest of the popular dairy-milk alternatives in saturated fat, at just 0.2 grams per cup. Almond milk is lower than soymilk in phytic acid, so you don't need to worry about reduced absorption of minerals. Almond milk also has none of the phytoestrogen concerns associated with soymilk.

Almond milk is high in vitamin E, but it's low in protein: One cup of almond milk contains just 1.3 grams of protein, compared to almost 8 grams in the same amount of dairy milk.

Other Options
You'll also find alternative "milks" made from cashews, rice, coconut, and even hemp. Among the latest entrants in the plant-milk craze is macadamia milk; it's richer and creamier because more of its calories come from fat (mostly unsaturated fat), but it provides no protein.

These beverages are all too new to have been extensively studied for possible health benefits, so check the Nutrition Facts label to see how they stack up against your current choices. Cashew milk, for example, which is made much like almond milk (and is sometimes combined with almond milk), contains only 25 calories in unsweetened form, no saturated fat, very little protein, and about 45 percent of your daily calcium. Cashew milk delivers even more vitamin E than almond milk.

Coconut milk in particular has been growing in popularity as part of the whole coconut health craze. Extracted from the grated flesh of ripe coconuts, canned coconut milk is popular in Asian and Caribbean cuisines; however, it is extremely high in saturated fat and calories. The thinned-down type of coconut milk sold in cartons in the dairy case is more similar to other milk alternatives, though it's still higher in saturated fat. Coconut milk contains less protein and calcium than almond, soy, cashew, or cow's milk but provides a creamy texture and light flavor.

If you like to drink cow's milk and prefer to pour it on your cereal, there's no health or nutrition reason to switch to any of these plant-based alternatives. Sticking with what you grew up with, in this case, is perfectly fine for healthy aging.

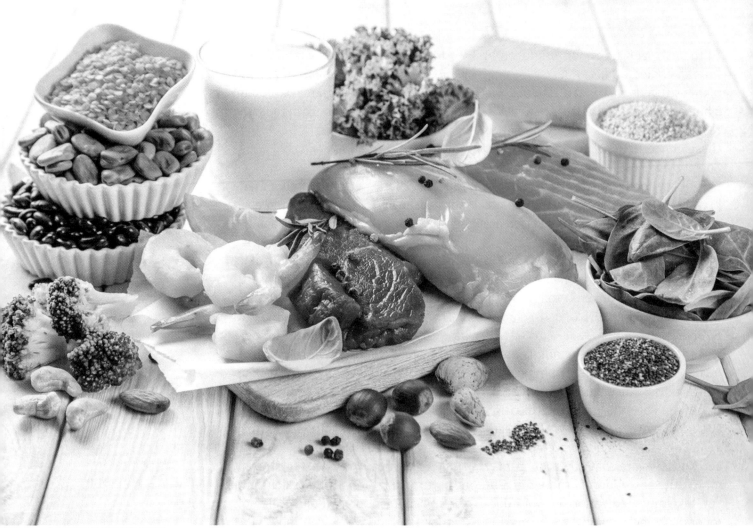

A variety of plant- and animal-sourced foods provide protein without the high saturated fat found in fatty cuts of meat and processed meats.

8 Protein Pros and Cons

With all the buzz about the protein-rich "Paleo," "keto," and low-carb diets, plus the marketing hype that's put protein claims on labels throughout the supermarket, you might be wondering if you need to boost your protein intake. Despite what you might hear from food companies, however, most Americans get plenty of protein—though the picture may be somewhat different for older individuals.

For one thing, older adults are more likely to be falling short on protein intake. "Although the RDA for protein is substantively the same for all adults, older adults tend to consume less protein than younger adults, primarily due to reduced energy needs," according to Paul F. Jacques, DSc, director of Tufts' HNRCA Nutritional Epidemiology Program. "Approximately one-third of adults over 50 years of age fail to meet the RDA for protein, and an estimated 10 percent of older women fail to meet even the lower Estimated Average Requirement for protein."

Your Protein Needs

The recommended dietary allowance (RDA) for protein is 46 grams for women and 56 grams for men, while the Daily Value percentage (% DV) used on nutrition labels is based on 50 grams. That's about as much protein as found in seven ounces of salmon or ground beef, one 6-ounce skinless chicken breast, or three cups of black beans.

However, experts say those general numbers should be adjusted according to a person's body weight. Most adults should aim for about 0.36 grams of protein per pound, so a person weighing 150 pounds needs about 54 grams of daily protein, while a 120-pound person requires 43 grams, and a 180-pound person needs 65 grams. Endurance runners and strength-training athletes need more—up to 0.8 grams per pound.

Many experts have argued that older adults should aim for more: 0.45 grams to 0.68 grams of protein per pound of body weight. For a 150-pound person, that translates to between 67.5 and 102 grams of protein daily—substantially more than the 50 grams used to calculate the % DV used in the Nutrition Facts panel.

Timing Matters

Even as scientists continue to study older adults' protein needs, evidence is mounting that the timing of that protein consumption may be important. A more even intake of protein throughout the day, rather than concentrating consumption at dinner, may provide maximum benefit.

One study found that spreading protein intake evenly throughout the day was associated with greater muscle mass and strength in 1,741 healthy adults, ages 67 to 84. Scientists commented, "Including one or more protein-rich foods at every meal is a simple way to stimulate your muscle-protein-building machinery, but it doesn't require a big portion—three to four ounces of fish or chicken breast, for example, is adequate. Breakfast is usually the meal that contains the least protein, so think about including at least one protein-rich food, such as dairy products, eggs, tofu, or quinoa."

Those findings echo an earlier clinical trial, in which eating extra protein at breakfast and lunch improved lean tissue mass in healthy older adults. Scientists randomly assigned participants, ages 55 to 66, to receive either protein

NEW FINDING

Extra Protein Fails to Benefit Older Men

Contrary to some earlier findings, a clinical trial reports that the Recommended Dietary Allowance (RDA) of protein may be sufficient to maintain muscle mass and function for older men. (The RDA is 0.36 grams of protein for each pound of body weight—about 58 grams for a 160-pound person and about 65 grams for a 180-pound person.) The study failed to demonstrate that increased intake of protein improves muscle mass, strength, or power as well as overall daily functioning. The trial involved 92 men age 65 and older who had moderate muscle-related limitations such as slower walking speed. At the start of the study, they were all consuming less than or just the right amount of their protein according to the RDA guidelines. The participants maintained their usual level of physical activity but avoided vigorous resistance and endurance exercise that could enhance muscle size or performance. The men were provided with pre-packaged, precisely formulated meals for six months and assigned randomly to eat meals containing the RDA for protein or meals with about 60 percent additional protein but the same number of calories. Men who consumed additional protein, compared with those eating the RDA level, saw no improvements in muscle performance, overall physical function, or lean body mass.

JAMA Internal Medicine, May 2018

supplements or a control compound at breakfast and lunch; the extra protein was split evenly between the two meals. Initially, most participants were consuming the majority of protein at dinner; adding the extra breakfast and lunch protein achieved a balance of about 30 percent of total protein intake at each meal. After 24 weeks, the participants who consumed roughly equal portions of protein throughout the day increased lean tissue mass by a significant amount—almost a pound on average—while those in the control group lost an average of more than a third of a pound.

According to Dr. Jacques, "Meeting a protein threshold of approximately 25 to 30 grams per meal represents a promising yet relatively unexplored dietary strategy to help maintain muscle mass and function in older adults."

Smart snacking also can add protein at times other than dinner. One study found that older adults who snack consume about 6 grams more protein daily than their non-snacking peers. An ounce of mixed nuts—about a handful—is a good snacking choice that provides 4.4

grams of protein. Another protein-rich option is a smoothie made with low-fat or nonfat yogurt.

Fending Off Frailty

An important reason why older adults in particular need to pay extra attention to protein is the role that protein plays in lean muscle mass. Sarcopenia, the gradual loss of lean muscle mass that can occur with aging, affects 15 percent of people older than age 65 and 50 percent of people older than age 80.

"Low muscle mass is a cause of poor muscle strength," says Martha Savaria Morris, PhD, a scientist in Tufts' HNRCA Nutritional Epidemiology Program. "One risk of having weak muscles is the inability to carry out activities of daily living and, consequently, a lack of independence. Another risk is falls, which often result in serious injury among older adults."

Research has shown that older adults who consume the most protein, including protein from animal as well as plant sources, are more likely to have the greatest muscle mass and strength. One study found that participants who scored highest in muscle mass and strength averaged substantially more than the RDA for protein: 93.4 grams daily for women and 101.1 grams for men.

The take-home message: Make sure you get enough protein from high-quality sources—perhaps even a bit more than recommended for your size—but don't go overboard. When you do consume protein, spread it out during the day rather than concentrating it at dinnertime.

Choosing Protein Sources

It's important to be selective when choosing sources of protein, because many less-healthy ingredients and nutrients often ride along with Americans' favorite protein foods. For example, topping your burger with bacon and cheese or digging into a slab of prime rib or other fatty meat will add a heaping helping of saturated fat. The Mediterranean-style diet offers a useful model of healthy protein sources; it includes more protein from fish and plant proteins and less from red meat. We'll look at these healthy protein powerhouses in the next chapter.

In any case, every gram of protein contains four calories, so if you incorporate more protein into your diet, be careful to avoid calorie overload. Rather

---

Protein by the Numbers

Getting enough protein doesn't have to mean packing away a double cheeseburger or tucking in to a full slab of ribs. Leaner cuts of red meat are good protein sources, as are poultry, fish, and plant foods (especially legumes). Here are some healthy foods high in protein:

Food	Protein	Food	Protein
Beef round steak (3 oz, cooked)	29 g	Rainbow trout (3 oz, cooked)	20 g
Soybeans (1 cup)	29 g	Halibut (3 oz, cooked)	19 g
Ricotta cheese (1 cup, part skim)	28 g	Veggie burger (3 oz)	19 g
Cottage cheese (1 cup, low-fat)	28 g	White beans (1 cup, cooked)	19 g
Chicken breast (3 oz, cooked)	27 g	Lentils (1 cup, cooked)	18 g
Pork tenderloin (3 oz, cooked)	26 g	Pinto beans (1 cup, cooked)	15 g
Turkey breast (3 oz, cooked)	25 g	Lima beans (1 cup, cooked)	15 g
Tuna, yellowfin (3 oz, cooked)	25 g	Chickpeas (1 cup, cooked)	15 g
Crab (3 oz, canned)	24 g	Greek yogurt, non-fat (5.3 oz, varies by brand)	12–15 g
Ground beef, 95% lean (3 oz, cooked)	22 g	Tofu, firm (3 oz, varies by brand)	7–10 g
Tuna, light (3 oz, canned in water)	22 g	Peanut butter (2 Tbsp)	9 g
Salmon (3 oz, cooked)	22 g	Green peas (1 cup, cooked)	8 g
Sardines (3 oz, canned)	21 g	Milk, low-fat (1 cup)	8 g
Chicken thigh (3 oz, cooked)	20 g	Egg, 1 whole, poached	7 g

Nuts and seeds also are high in protein, but, because of their calorie density, they should be consumed in smaller quantities. A quarter-cup of almonds, for example, contains 7.5 grams of protein and 207 calories. A quarter-cup of pumpkin seeds has 8.8 grams of protein and 169 calories. The same holds for nut butters: Two tablespoons of peanut butter provide 7.1 grams of protein and 191 calories.

than simply adding more protein to your regular diet, substitute lower-calorie foods containing protein for less healthy food choices, such as refined carbohydrates, fried foods, or sugary desserts.

On the plus side, some protein sources contribute other desirable nutrients as a bonus. For example, salmon and some other fish provide omega-3 fatty acids that may benefit your heart and brain as you age. Beans, peas, lentils, nuts, and seeds deliver dietary fiber as well as protein. We'll take a closer look at seafood and plant sources of protein in the next chapter.

Causes for Caution

Another reason not to overdo your protein intake, despite the marketing and fad-diet hype, is concern that too much might contribute to certain medical conditions. A 2018 study concluded that middle-aged men who ate higher amounts of protein-rich meats and dairy foods had a slightly higher risk of heart failure than those who ate less protein. Protein from fish and eggs was not associated with heart failure, however.

The association between high protein intake and heart failure found in this study was small—but this study serves as a reminder that dietary intake in excess of recommendations can have unintended consequences.

If you have certain medical conditions, you may be advised to limit your protein intake. For example, people with chronic kidney disease should avoid high-protein diets, which may further damage kidney function. Diets high in protein may increase the risk of kidney stones, even in those with otherwise healthy kidneys.

And patients with gout should consult their physicians about protein intake. Many protein sources, including red meat, poultry, and fish, contain purines, which the body breaks down to form uric acid, the cause of the painful swelling in gout.

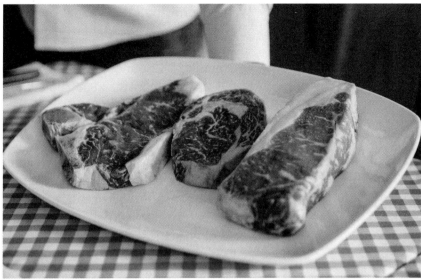

© Artitwpd | Dreamstime

Some cuts of beef are very high in saturated fat; the higher the fat content, the more "marbling" (streaks and flecks of visible fat) in the meat.

Protein from Red Meat

Red meat is a prime source of protein in the U.S. diet, but health concerns have Americans loving it a little less lately. A study by the Natural Resources Defense Council reported that Americans reduced their intake of beef by nearly one-fifth between 2005 and 2014. Pork consumption also fell, though not as drastically.

Beef and pork, along with veal, lamb, and goat meat, are considered "red" meat because they contain more of a protein called myoglobin. Found in the muscle tissue of almost all mammals, myoglobin binds iron and oxygen. According to the USDA definition, all meats obtained from mammals are considered red meat, as opposed to "white" meat obtained from fish and poultry.

Red Meat Risks

Red meat, it's true, is a concentrated source of protein and other healthy nutrients. A 3.5-ounce portion of 90%-lean ground beef delivers 20 grams of protein, along with significant amounts of niacin, vitamin B_{12}, iron, zinc, and selenium. However, that portion of beef contains 10 grams of saturated fat, which is more than half the total recommended daily limit. Beef cuts with a higher fat content, including many varieties of steak, push the calorie and saturated fat numbers even higher—as do the larger portion sizes typically found in restaurants. For example, a 12-ounce ribeye steak tips the scales at more than 800 calories and more than 20 grams of saturated fat.

We've already seen why it's important to limit intakes of processed red meats, such as bacon, ham, salami, and sausage: Studies have consistently linked consumption of processed red meats to increased risks of mortality, cardiovascular disease, and cancer. Findings for unprocessed red meat have been less conclusive. Nonetheless, an expert panel of 22 scientists from the World Health Organization's International Agency for Research on Cancer concluded that red meat probably contributes to colon, prostate, and pancreatic cancer risk.

However, even the association between red meat consumption and cancer risk may be complex. It is possible, for example, that high-temperature cooking of red meat, which forms possible carcinogens such as heterocyclic amines, polycyclic aromatic hydrocarbons, and advanced glycation end-products, may be responsible for increased cancer risk, rather than the meat itself. So, your slow-cooked brisket or pork shoulder may be safer than those steaks or chops sizzling on the grill.

Expert Advice

Most nutrition experts suggest eating less red meat. The Dietary Guidelines Advisory Committee, a group of nutrition experts tasked with assisting in the update of those guidelines, recommended that a healthy dietary pattern should be "lower in red and processed meats." While no longer emphasizing limiting total fat consumption, the expert panel did focus on limiting foods high in saturated fat—including many cuts of red meat. Their report also noted that a diet that emphasizes more plant foods and less meat is "more health promoting and is associated with less environmental impact."

The resulting 2015-2020 *Dietary Guidelines for Americans* (*DGA*) similarly recommends eating a variety of protein foods, including lean meats along with seafood, poultry, eggs, legumes (beans and peas), nuts, seeds, and soy products. But Dariush Mozaffarian, MD, DrPH, dean of Tufts' Friedman School, notes that this recommendation was watered down from the original expert panel's "strong, explicit recommendations that Americans should eat less of two major food groups: red and processed meats, and refined grains. The harms of these foods, and the need to reduce them, was a major focus. Notably, the scientific panel only advised sensible reductions—not elimination—of meats and refined grains; they did not say that all Americans should become vegans, or eat only quinoa. Yet, the final *DGA* ignores (for meats) or hides (for refined grains) this strong, sound advice."

A review of the scientific evidence authored by Dr. Mozaffarian identified dietary priorities for cardiovascular and metabolic health. He concluded that individuals should limit their consumption of processed meat to no more than one serving per week and have no more than one to two servings of unprocessed red meats per week. Keep in mind that one serving is generally 3.5 ounces of meat—not the platefuls of ribs or double-patty burgers so many Americans commonly consume.

To sum up, eat small servings of red meat once or twice a week (if you enjoy it) and have processed meat only occasionally. When you do cook meat, avoid charring and high-heat cooking. Low, slow, moist braises—which are perfect for more affordable cuts—may minimize the formation of carcinogenic compounds while allowing much of the fat to cook out.

What About Eggs?

Eggs are another favorite—and affordable—protein source, but the evidence on eggs and health is more mixed than for red and processed meats. Because the yolks are high in dietary cholesterol, eggs have long been viewed as unhealthy. But experts have discovered that dietary cholesterol plays a much smaller part in raising unhealthy blood cholesterol levels than previously believed, and now eggs—in moderation—are back on the menu. Both the American Heart Association and the *DGA* say it's no longer necessary to strictly recommend limiting dietary cholesterol to 300 milligrams daily for healthy people. (One large egg contains about 186 milligrams of cholesterol.) As science continues to sort out the health impacts of eggs, however, it's wise not to go overboard; unlimited dietary cholesterol might not be the best advice for everyone.

Eggs deliver many important vitamins and minerals, including vitamins B_{12} and D, choline, selenium, and iodine, and are an exceptional source of protein. The 7 grams of protein in a large egg contain all of the essential amino acids you need to obtain from your diet; in fact, the World Health Organization uses eggs as the standard for evaluating the biological value of protein in all other foods.

Egg yolks are a source of lutein and zeaxanthin, caroteinoids that help protect your eyes against conditions such as macular degeneration. Although the amounts in eggs are relatively small, Tufts research has shown that the carotenoids in egg yolks may be more readily available for use by the body than those from other foods.

The nutrients in eggs are split between the yolk and the white, with a little more than half the protein found in the white and all of the saturated fat in the yolk. The yolk also contains all of the carotenoids and most of the calories.

Liquid egg substitutes are made from the white only, so they have fewer calories and no fat or cholesterol. Some varieties have been fortified with vitamins and minerals to make up for the nutrients found in the yolk; check the ingredients list to see if any nutrients have been added.

Cracking the Facts About Eggs

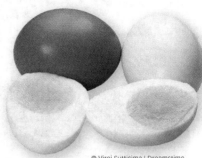
© Viroj Suttisima | Dreamstime

- Don't worry about shell color. White and brown eggs are nutritionally the same. Shell color is determined by the breed of hen, with brown and red hens laying brown eggs.

- Egg grading is not determined by freshness, but by factors such as the quality of the white, absence of yolk defects, and shell cleanness and integrity. In general, however, an "AA" egg will stay fresh longer than an egg graded "A."

- Organic standards require hens to have access to the outdoors. In terms of nutrition and health, independent reviews generally report no significant differences between organic and conventional eggs.

- Salmonella contamination of eggs from chickens is impossible to detect by simple observation and is unrelated to eggs' freshness. Raw, soft-cooked, and "sunny-side-up" eggs are riskier; if you prefer such preparations, consider pasteurized eggs, which are nutritionally identical. (You can also pasteurize eggs in the shell using those popular sous vide cookers, at 135 degrees for two hours; refrigerate and consume within a few days.) Because of the risk of cross-contamination, wash all surfaces exposed to raw egg, much as you would with raw chicken.

- Store eggs, unwashed, with the pointier end down in their carton on a shelf inside the refrigerator. Avoid the fridge door, where temperatures vary more.

- Eggs' expiration date is calculated based on when they were packaged (maximum 30 days from packaging to expiration), not when they were laid. The time between laying and packaging can be as little as a few days or as much as a few weeks. Eggs can generally be consumed even after the expiration date; the USDA says raw eggs in the shell can be safely stored in the fridge for up to five weeks.

- Hard-boiled eggs, even unpeeled, spoil faster than raw eggs because the water removes a protective coating and exposes the shell's pores to bacteria. Refrigerate unpeeled and eat within a week.

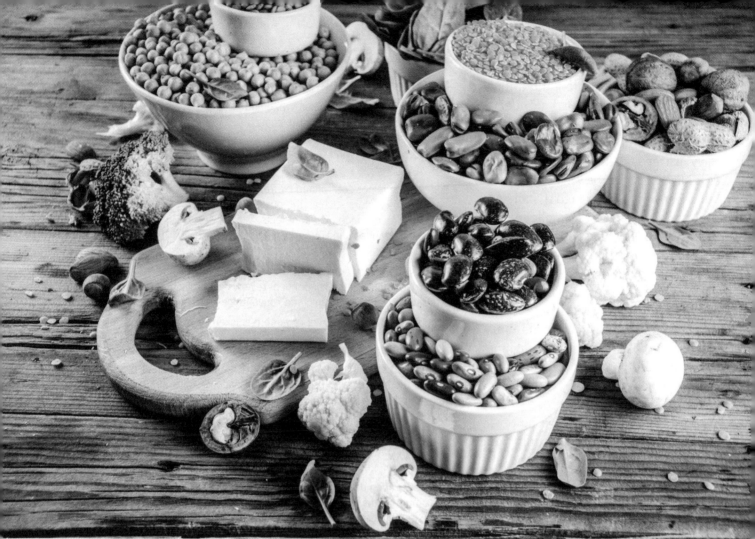

Fish, beans, peas, lentils, nuts, seeds, and soy foods provide protein. Some of these foods are high in fiber, and some are good sources of healthy, unsaturated fats.

9 Top Protein Picks

Animal foods, including meats, poultry, eggs, and dairy products, currently provide the bulk of Americans' protein—and most people consume much more than they need from less healthy sources such as red and processed meat. On the other hand, many people fall short in reaching recommendations for twice-weekly servings of fish. In addition to providing protein with fewer calories than most meat, many varieties of seafood contain heart-healthy omega-3 fatty acids. Minimally processed plant foods that contain protein also provide valuable vitamins, minerals, fiber, and phytochemicals associated with a healthy dietary pattern. An easy, tasty way to improve your diet is to exchange some meat protein for seafood and plant proteins.

Protein from Seafood

A three-ounce serving of fish provides 30 to 40 percent of your daily protein requirements. And fish contains less connective tissue than meat or poultry, so it's easier to digest. Fish is also a natural source of B_{12} and other B vitamins you may be lacking. You'll get some vitamin D and minerals from fish, too, including selenium, zinc, iron, and iodine.

The *Dietary Guidelines* and nutrition experts recommend eating fatty fish, such as salmon, mackerel, herring, and sardines, because they are high in omega-3 fatty acids (notably, docosahexaenoic acid, or DHA, and eicosapentaenoic acid, or EPA). However, leaner varieties also are healthy choices, especially if you use smart cooking methods.

Fish that are lower in fat, such as cod, pollock, haddock, and flounder, also are lower in calories, with less than 120 calories per three-ounce cooked serving versus 175 calories for a similar-sized portion of salmon. Like all fish, lean varieties are low in saturated fat (unless they are breaded or battered and fried).

Don't obsess over the omega-3 content of specific fish varieties. Eating whatever fish you prefer—even the omnipresent tilapia—is a smart protein choice. Tufts' Alice H. Lichtenstein, DSc, points out, "Fish offers heart-healthy omega-3 fatty acids and is low in calories and saturated fat. Tilapia happens to be lower in fat than some other fish, so it has less of all types of fatty acids, including omega-3. Tilapia is, however, more affordable than most other fish in the market today."

Eating more fish might have some surprising benefits beyond the heart-health effects of omega-3s—such as easing the joint pain and swelling of rheumatoid arthritis (RA). In a 2018 study, RA patients were grouped by fish consumption—less than one serving a month, one a month, one to two a week, and more than two servings a week. A "disease activity score" was used to rate the severity of RA symptoms based on pain and swelling. After controlling for other factors including use of fish oil supplements, the study found that RA pain and swelling declined as fish consumption increased.

Cooking Methods Are Key

One advantage of substituting fish for other protein sources such as beef and pork is what you're *not* getting as much of: the calories, saturated fat, and high sodium often found in entrées replaced by fish. When you're eating broiled salmon or baked cod, you aren't chowing down on pizza, burgers, hot dogs, or fried chicken.

Much of that healthy advantage vanishes, however, when you bread and fry fish or slather it in butter or rich sauces. One study found that women who ate fish most often were at lower risk of heart failure—but that finding applied only to eating baked or broiled fish. Fried fish was actually associated with an increased risk of heart failure. Other research has linked fried fish to a higher risk of stroke. Similarly, while data from the Cardiovascular Health Study linked weekly intake of broiled or baked fish with greater brain volume in MRI scans, those who ate fried fish saw no brain benefit.

Other healthy ways to cook fish include steaming, poaching, and grilling at moderate temperatures. Because fish tends to stick to the grill, consider using aluminum grill toppers or cooking your fish in foil packets or parchment paper with veggies and herbs.

Shopping Basics

Keep in mind that similar varieties of fish can be substituted in recipes. Just be mindful of the basic characteristics of the fish that's called for—flaky, firm, steak-like, fatty, or lean.

If you're concerned about sustainability, check the Seafood Watch guide at www.seafoodwatch.org.

Mercury contamination is an important concern for women who are pregnant or planning to become pregnant, but most older individuals can choose the fish they prefer in moderation without much concern about mercury. Eating a wide variety of seasonably available fresh or frozen fish is the best way to get the benefits of seafood with few downsides.

Fish Favorites

Although the earth's oceans, lakes, and streams are home to more than 27,000 types of fish, about 30 species make up the majority of fish found in America's supermarkets. Here are some tips for choosing and using some of the most popular varieties.

NEW FINDING

Older Adults Protected by Omega-3s

Here's another reason to have fish tonight: A study has found an association between higher levels of omega-3 polyunsaturated fatty acids in the blood and healthy aging. The research analyzed data from 2,622 U.S. adults, measuring levels of omega-3s at three points over 13 years. Consistently having higher levels of omega-3 such as those found in seafood was associated with an 18 percent decrease in risk of developing cardiovascular disease, cancer, lung disease, and severe chronic kidney disease during the study period. These findings suggest that eating more seafood could increase the likelihood of healthy aging in older adults. The alpha-linolenic omega-3s found in plants were not significantly associated with healthy aging.
British Medical Journal, October 17, 2018

Don't Overlook Lean Fish

Lean fish may be lower in omega-3s than fatty fish, but they do contain some omega-3s, as well as protein and vitamin B$_{12}$, and they're generally lower in calories than fatty fish. Here are some nutrition numbers for varieties of lean fish.

TYPE OF FISH (PER 3 oz COOKED)	CALORIES	PROTEIN	VITAMIN B$_{12}$	TOTAL OMEGA-3s
Cod	89	19g	0.9mcg	142mg
Flounder	73	13g	1.11mcg	334mg
Grouper	100	21g	0.6mcg	265mg
Haddock	76	17g	1.8mcg	141mg
Mahi mahi	93	20g	1.1mcg	128mg
Pollock	100	21g	3.13mcg	484mg
Rockfish	93	19g	1.35mcg	316mg
Snapper	109	22g	3.0mcg	292mg
Tilapia	111	23g	1.6mcg	165mg

Source: USDA National Nutrient Database; grams = g, milligrams = mg, micrograms = mcg

Catfish. No longer the "muddy"-flavored bottom-feeder you might remember, catfish is now second only to tilapia in aquaculture popularity. Whether it's fresh or frozen, look for farmed catfish that are white to off-white. Four ounces of cooked catfish contain just 119 calories but more than 20 grams of protein, along with 607 milligrams of omega-3s.

Cod. Wild cod is available year-round; small, young fish also may be called "scrod" (a term also applied to haddock). Flaky and mild in flavor, cod is versatile and can be used in any recipe calling for mild whitefish. A 4-ounce serving of cooked Pacific cod has only 96 calories while delivering 21 grams of protein. Cod is low in fat of all types, with 250 milligrams of omega-3s in 4 ounces.

Flounder. Flounder has sweet, delicate flesh that rewards gentle cooking. It's also sold as "sole" or "lemon sole" or "fluke." (North America produces no true species of sole; only imported "Dover sole" is actually sole.) A 4-ounce portion of cooked flounder has just 97 calories, but 17 grams of protein and 287 milligrams of omega-3s.

Haddock. A popular choice for frying in fish and chips, haddock (also sometimes called "scrod") can be prepared in healthy ways like other lean fish with firm, mild flesh. There are 102 calories and 23 grams of protein in 4 ounces of cooked haddock, 233 milligrams of omega-3s.

Halibut. Lower in fat than other steak-style fish, halibut can be baked, poached, or cooked on skewers, but keep a close eye on it, as it easily can be overcooked. Look for halibut with almost translucent white flesh. Fresh halibut is available year-round but is most abundant from March to September. A 4-ounce serving of cooked halibut contains 126 calories and 25 grams of protein. Though halibut is a relatively lean fish, it delivers a significant amount of omega-3s—592 milligrams per 4 ounces.

Mahi Mahi. Also called "dorado" or "dolphinfish" (but unrelated to the dolphin, which is a mammal), this Hawaiian favorite is increasingly available in mainland supermarkets. Mahi mahi has firm, white flesh and is best prepared simply, such as broiled or grilled. Four ounces of cooked mahi mahi contain only 126 calories but a significant 27 grams of protein, plus 177 milligrams of omega-3s.

Pollock. This member of the cod family can be found as fillets or steaks, fresh or frozen, sold under a befuddling variety of names including "blue cod," "blue snapper," "Boston bluefish," "coalfish," and "saithe." If you've purchased imitation crab products ("surimi"), you've probably eaten pollock without even knowing it. Its flesh is firm, delicate, and slightly sweet, and it can be substituted in recipes for cod. A 4-ounce portion of cooked pollock has 126 calories, nearly 27 grams of protein, and 503 milligrams of omega-3s.

Salmon. After shrimp and tuna, salmon is America's third most-consumed seafood. A 4-ounce portion of cooked salmon contains about 29 grams of protein and between 177 and 236 calories, depending on the type of salmon.

Salmon is known for its omega-3 content. In general, omega-3 levels are highest in salmon species that swim in the coldest waters, such as king salmon, because these fats stay liquid at frigid temperatures and serve as a sort of "antifreeze" for the fish, as well as a main energy source. Wild-caught salmon species—king (also called chinook), coho (or silver), sockeye, chum, and pink (primarily sold canned)—account for about a third of all U.S. salmon consumption. Fish sold as "Atlantic salmon" is actually farm-raised.

If you can't find fresh salmon, check the freezer section. Flash-frozen salmon is as nutritious as fresh and keeps for about four months in the freezer. Canned salmon is not only an environmentally sound choice, but, if it is canned with bones, it delivers a bonus of calcium.

Swordfish. Swordfish is at its fresh peak in summer months, although it is available frozen year-round. It has a meaty texture that lends itself to almost any cooking method. Four ounces of cooked swordfish contain 195 calories and 27 grams of protein, along with 924 milligrams of omega-3s. However, swordfish ranks as one of the fish highest in mercury content, so enjoy it only occasionally.

Tilapia. Popular for its easy preparation and lean flesh that remains moist when cooked, tilapia is the most commonly sold farmed fish in the U.S. Look for fillets that are white or pinkish-white. Tilapia can be baked, broiled, steamed, or grilled (using an aluminum grill topper). A 4-ounce serving of cooked tilapia has 139 calories, 28 grams of protein, and 246 milligrams of omega-3s.

Trout. Available in several varieties, farmed or wild-caught, as fillets as well as whole fish, trout is related to salmon and similarly rich in omega-3s, with 1,196 milligrams of omega-3s per 4 ounces. Preparation options are equally varied, and steelhead trout (rainbow trout that migrate to the ocean) is interchangeable with salmon in fillet recipes. Nutrition numbers vary by trout species; 4 ounces of cooked fish provide between 170 and 215 calories and 26 to 30 grams of protein.

Tuna. A meaty fish suitable for most cooking preparations (be careful not to overcook it, however), tuna is sold fresh or frozen as steaks, as well as canned. Tuna nutrition numbers vary by species: Four ounces of cooked skipjack tuna, for example, contain 150 calories, 32 grams of protein, and 301 milligrams of omega-3s; skipjack also is sold canned as "light" tuna. Four ounces of canned albacore ("white") tuna, packed in water, contain 145 calories, 27 grams of protein, and 1,064 milligrams of omega-3 fatty acids.

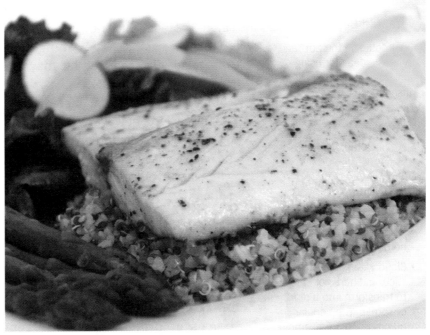

Mahi mahi is a firm, white fish that can be baked, broiled, or grilled; serve with a whole grain, a salad, and a vegetable for a healthy meal that's packed with nutrients.

If you enjoy canned tuna as tuna "salad," go easy on the high-calorie, high-fat additions. Try making your tuna salad with reduced-fat mayo or even with low-fat yogurt.

Tuna is also a popular ingredient in sushi. Be aware, however, that the FDA advises older adults, pregnant women, and people with compromised immune systems to avoid raw fish, which may contain harmful bacteria or parasites.

Protein from Plants

You may be hesitant to count on plants to meet some or all of your protein needs because of concerns about getting "complete" protein. All animal sources of protein (including seafood, eggs, and dairy) deliver adequate amounts of all nine "essential" amino acids—the building blocks of protein—that the body can't make itself. Foods that meet this requirement are called "complete" proteins. Grains (with the notable exception of quinoa) are usually not an adequate source of the amino acids lysine and isoleucine, so they are not complete proteins.

According to Diane McKay, PhD, the Tufts consulting editor for this report, "All plant-based foods have most of the nine essential amino acids, but in some foods, they are present in particularly low amounts; these are called limiting amino acids. If you eat enough of these foods, however, you will be able to get enough of that limiting amino acid to help your body make proteins."

You don't have to obtain all of the essential amino acids at a single meal; it's the balance over a whole day that matters. The importance of "complete" proteins, however, is why people often eat rice with beans—together, they deliver all of the essential amino acids, as do peanut butter plus whole-grain bread.

Dr. McKay offers some examples of other combinations of plant-based foods that will help you reach the amount of the limiting amino acids without having to eat a large amount of any single plant food (or pig out on meat). One smart strategy is to combine grains (preferably whole) or nuts/seeds with beans and legumes. That's because the grains and nuts/seeds are limited in the amino acid lysine but are rich in methionine, while beans and legumes are low in methionine but rich in lysine. So consider these combo plates:

- Red beans and brown rice
- Black beans and corn tortillas
- Hummus and pita bread
- Nut butter and whole-grain bread
- Peas and pasta
- Bean soup and whole-grain crackers

We've already looked at some of the many healthy, tasty options in whole grains, which contribute protein as well as fiber and other nutrients. Other plant-protein sources, as suggested by the list above, include legumes, nuts, and seeds.

Legumes Do Double Duty

Legumes, which include beans, peas, and lentils, are the only food type that appears in the USDA's MyPlate recommendations in two different categories—the Vegetable Group and the Protein Foods Group.

When choosing beans, you can select whatever types—kidney, white, garbanzo, cannellini, black, lima, pinto, navy—most appeal to you, since, nutritionally, there are few important differences. Beans deliver between 6 and 8.5 grams of protein per cooked half-cup serving, as well as soluble fiber (5 to 9.5 grams total fiber per serving), which can help improve your body's blood cholesterol levels.

Consuming beans has been associated with better cholesterol levels and a reduced risk of death from heart disease. The fiber in beans also may help encourage the growth of healthy bacteria in the lower digestive tract, which could be a reason some research has linked bean consumption to a lower risk of colon cancer.

Beans' combination of fiber plus protein makes them a good choice for blood-sugar balance and regulation. The American Diabetes Association lists beans as a "diabetes superfood," noting, "Beans do contain carbohydrates, but a half cup also provides as much protein as an ounce of meat without the saturated fat."

Beans are also high in manganese, which is important to the body's enzyme reactions. And beans provide thiamin (vitamin B_1), which is required for the synthesis of acetylcholine, a key neurotransmitter essential to the brain's memory functions; low acetylcholine levels are associated with dementia and Alzheimer's disease.

Unlike most vegetables, which lose nutrients in lengthy, high-temperature cooking, dried beans require such cooking to be edible. Canned, pre-cooked beans are equally nutritious; buy reduced-sodium or no-salt-added varieties and drain and rinse thoroughly.

Varieties of peas, including black-eyed peas, chickpeas, and split peas, are similar to beans in protein and fiber content, as are lentils of all types (green, red, and yellow). These protein-rich plant foods are especially good choices for making hearty soups and stews. Another plus is that all legumes are budget-friendly, costing far less than most animal sources of high-quality protein.

Noshing On Nuts

The findings keep coming demonstrating the many health benefits of eating nuts. Although nuts are calorie-dense, they also are nutrient-dense, including protein, and most healthy eating patterns recommend eating several servings each week.

"Nuts are tiny nutritional powerhouses, which taste as good as they are good for you," says Tufts expert Jeffrey Blumberg, PhD. "Nuts are an excellent source of vitamin E and magnesium, nutrients many Americans don't get enough of. Individuals consuming nuts also have higher intakes of folate, beta-carotene, vitamin K, lutein plus zeaxanthin, phosphorus, copper, selenium, potassium, and zinc per 1,000 calories."

Nuts are rich in unsaturated fats, but their cholesterol benefits exceed what would be expected from heart-healthy fats alone. Nuts provide phytosterols and flavonoids (types of phytonutrients) and dietary fiber, which also are likely to contribute to cardiovascular health.

Putting Nuts to the Test. Multiple studies have demonstrated cardiovascular benefits from eating nuts, especially improvements in cholesterol levels and blood-vessel function. A Tufts review of 61 prior trials found that nut intake lowered total cholesterol, unhealthy LDL cholesterol, triglycerides, and lipoproteins (particles that transport fats through the body).

In other study findings based on three large health studies spanning more than 30 years, eating nuts was associated with better cardiovascular health. After controlling for other cardiovascular risk factors, the more nuts people consumed, the lower their risk for coronary heart disease and cardiovascular disease. Even eating less than a single one-ounce serving of nuts per week was associated with a 9 percent lower risk of heart attack and stroke and a 12 percent lower risk of CHD, compared to eating zero nuts. Those apparent benefits jumped to 14 percent and 20 percent among people who ate a one-ounce serving of nuts five times a week.

Nuts also have antioxidant and anti-inflammatory properties, and they have been found to improve insulin resistance, which is important for the prevention of diabetes. The large PREDIMED

Going Nuts

Start incorporating nuts into your daily diet as a substitute for less-healthy snacks. You can also use nuts as part of other dishes, replacing some meat, cream, or other ingredients. Here are some ideas:

- Combine nuts with herbs such as basil or parsley, along with olive oil, to make pesto.
- Top salads with nuts instead of croutons or cheese.
- Add nuts to steamed vegetables or stir-fry entrées.
- Use nuts to add crunch to whole-grain dishes.
- Thicken sauces with ground nuts.
- Sprinkle nuts on yogurt.
- Include nuts in homemade granola.
- Use nuts in stir-fry dishes in place of some of the meat.

The downside of nuts' high unsaturated fat content is that it makes them prone to spoiling and going rancid. To prolong edibility, keep nuts in an airtight container in your refrigerator or a sealed plastic bag in your freezer; don't store near foods whose odors might be absorbed by the nuts. If you buy large quantities of nuts at a warehouse club, separate into smaller amounts and bag using a vacuum sealer; because almost all the air is sucked out, unopened vacuum-sealed nuts will stay fresh on your pantry shelf for months.

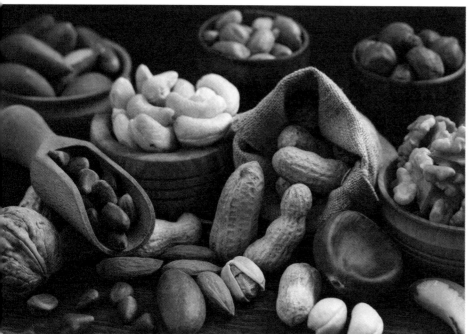
© Andrey Maslakov | Dreamstime

Clinical studies have found links between eating nuts and having a lower risk of heart disease, heart attack, stroke, and diabetes.

observational study found that a Mediterranean-style diet supplemented with nuts was associated with lower incidence of type 2 diabetes.

People who eat more nuts may even live longer. An analysis of data from more than 350,000 participants reported an association between regular nut consumption and reduced mortality risk. Eating a serving of nuts—about an ounce, or a medium handful—every day was associated with a 39 percent lower risk of cardiovascular mortality and a 27 percent lower risk of all-cause mortality.

Nuts and Weight. A small handful of nuts contains up to 200 calories, but people who eat them experience less weight gain over time, according to a 10-country European study of more than 370,000 people. Compared with people who didn't eat nuts, those consuming more than one serving (one ounce) per week had a 10 percent lower increase in body weight. This study doesn't prove eating nuts reduces weight gain, but it does suggest that eating nuts regularly may not make it harder to stay trim.

Another study found an inverse relationship between eating nuts and weight gain; nuts ranked second only to yogurt as a food linked to losing weight. And in general, studies have found that people whose diets are higher in nuts typically don't weigh more.

What could explain these findings? Some research suggests that not all of the calories in nuts may be absorbed by the body. Nuts also tend to be filling since they contain both fiber and protein, which may result in lower consumption of other foods, especially other snack foods that may be high in calories, added sugar, sodium, and/or saturated fat.

It's always smarter to substitute a healthy choice like nuts for less-healthy options such as chips and cookies. Dr. Blumberg notes, "Nuts are part of the USDA MyPlate portion of protein, so you can also think about substituting them for a serving or less of red meat."

Picking Nuts. At the supermarket, choose whatever variety of nuts you like best, since the nutrient profiles of nuts are more similar than different. Your choices also can include peanuts, since these legumes have nutritional properties similar to tree nuts. Here are some nutritional highlights of various types of nuts:

- **Almonds** top all tree nuts per ounce in protein, fiber, calcium, vitamin E, niacin, and riboflavin.
- **Brazil** nuts are among the richest dietary sources of selenium and are also high in magnesium.
- **Cashews** are the tree nuts highest in iron, copper, and zinc.
- **Hazelnuts,** also called filberts, are good sources of vitamin E, manganese, and copper.
- **Macadamia nuts** contain the most calories and fat of all nuts, but most of the fat is of the healthy monounsaturated variety.
- **Peanuts** are high in fiber, vitamin E, magnesium, folate, and niacin.

- **Pecans** are packed with antioxidants and vitamin E.
- **Pine nuts,** also known as piñon, pinoli, or pignoli, are second only to walnuts in polyunsaturated fat content and provide more than 100 percent of the recommended daily intake of manganese in one serving.
- **Pistachios,** the only tree nuts that can be roasted in their shells, have the most potassium and vitamin B_6.
- **Walnuts** are the only nut rich in alpha-linolenic acid (ALA), the plant form of omega-3 fatty acids.

Tiny Seeds, Big Nutrition

Protein-packed snack and ingredient options also include seeds, such as sunflower, sesame, pumpkin, flax, and even hemp and chia seeds (as in "chia pets"). Like walnuts, many varieties of seeds contain ALA, which research has shown can help protect blood vessels from inflammatory damage and lower the risk of atherosclerosis.

In addition to being high in ALA, flaxseed also may confer blood-pressure benefits. In one Canadian study, participants who received 30 grams of milled flaxseed (the equivalent of three heaping tablespoons) daily had significantly lower blood pressure readings than participants who didn't receive flaxseed. On average, their systolic pressure (the top number) dropped 10 mmHg, while diastolic pressure (the bottom number) fell 7 mmHg. Those changes, researchers noted, were superior to other dietary interventions and similar to what is often achieved by prescription medication.

Whole flaxseed isn't broken down in your digestive tract, so you'll need ground flaxseed to get maximum nutritional benefits. It's easy to grind flaxseed in a spice or coffee grinder, or you can buy flaxseed that has been ground already. Flax meal and milled flaxseed are the same as ground flaxseed.

Seeds also provide fiber, protein, and a variety of phytonutrients. Whether you snack on pumpkin or sunflower seeds or sprinkle hemp or chia seeds into yogurt, you can improve your nutrient intake by adding seeds to your dietary pattern.

As these examples show, you have many options for getting the protein your body needs—and not all your protein sources need to be served on a bun or carved with a steak knife.

NEW FINDING

Walnuts Could Improve Cholesterol

The evidence keeps adding up that nuts, once considered a snack indulgence, are good for you. Now a review and analysis reports that eating walnuts could improve blood lipid levels (cholesterol and triglycerides)—without causing weight gain or increasing blood pressure. Scientists analyzed data from 26 controlled trials evaluating the effects of walnut consumption on blood lipids and other cardiovascular risk factors. Participants who ate more walnuts had a 3.3 percent greater reduction in total blood cholesterol, a 3.7 percent greater reduction in LDL cholesterol, and a 5.5 percent greater reduction in triglyceride concentrations compared with those who did not eat walnuts. Weight and blood pressure in the walnut-enriched-diet groups were not significantly different from those of the controls.

American Journal of Clinical Nutrition, July 2018

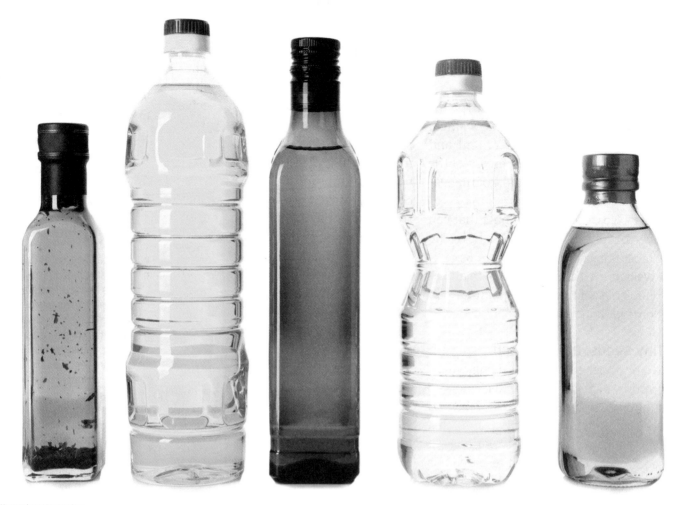

Make most of your fat unsaturated fat—the type tied to health benefits—and limit animal-sourced foods high in saturated fat.

10 Fresh Thinking on Fats

We've already touched on how the scientific consensus has changed when it comes to fats: Focus on the types of fats in your diet rather than worrying about total fat intake (except as one way of cutting calories). The last report from the Dietary Guidelines Advisory Committee (DGAC) notably omitted any upper limit on total fat consumption, as did the 2015-2020 *Dietary Guidelines for Americans*. The DGAC noted that reducing total fat intake by substituting carbohydrates does not reduce cardiovascular risk, concluding, "Dietary advice should put the emphasis on optimizing types of dietary fat and not reducing total fat."

Adjust Your Attitude Toward Fat

If you're like most Americans, however, according to a Gallup survey, one of your goals for a healthy diet is to limit consumption of all fats. Though that's no longer scientifically sound advice, you can hardly be blamed for this way of thinking. After all, for years, we were told to cut back on fats, and food manufacturers created many "low-fat" products, from cookies to salad dressings, that appeared on supermarket shelves. That low-fat craze turned out to be counterproductive, leading people to substitute refined carbohydrates for dietary fats (hence, the DGAC's caution about choosing carbs in place of fats). You might think of this as the "Snack-Wells" effect—swapping cookies and other sugary snacks for higher-fat foods. The result was a runaway obesity epidemic: Between 1980 and 2000, obesity rates among U.S. adults doubled.

The Nutrition Facts panel on food labels similarly reflected this outdated thinking: It still singled out "calories from fat," suggesting this is something important to limit, and percentages were based on a 1980 recommendation of 30 percent of calories from fat, or 65 grams per day. The FDA's definition of "healthy" as a claim allowed on packaging still includes a requirement that a product be low not just in saturated fat but also in total fat, although that's also now under review.

How Fats Affect You

It's true that fat is a concentrated source of calories, with 9 calories per gram of fat compared to 4 calories per gram of protein or carbohydrate. That's why limiting fat intake seemed like a sound strategy for preventing obesity.

Calories aside, however, not all fats affect the body the same way. Although the role and mechanism of saturated fats in contributing to unhealthy blood cholesterol levels continues to be a subject of debate and research, recent studies clearly support the health benefits of substituting healthy mono- and polyunsaturated fats for saturated fats. Those healthy fats include the omega-3 fats found in fish, which were discussed in the previous chapter. Choosing healthy unsaturated fats is more beneficial than simply limiting your intake of total fats.

A classic example is the avocado, a plant food high in total fat that some people avoided for that reason. Most of the fat in avocados is unsaturated, however, and studies have shown that including avocados in the diet is associated with better heart health.

Complex Chemistry

Dietary fats, including those found in cooking oils, are classified as saturated, monounsaturated, and polyunsaturated fats based on their fundamental chemistry. Most foods that contain fat contain both types of unsaturated fat as well as saturated fat; those from animal sources,

such as butter and lard, as well as tropical sources such as coconut and palm oil, tend to be higher in saturated fat.

Common vegetable oils, as well as the fats in meat and dairy, contain a mix of different types of fatty acids. Olive oil is mostly oleic acid (a monounsaturated fat), for example, while safflower oil is rich in linoleic acid (a polyunsaturated fat). Coconut oil is high in lauric acid, a type of saturated fat.

Different types of fats can affect your entrée choices, too. Animal products such as meat tend to be high in saturated fat, so substituting fish high in unsaturated omega-3s can improve your overall fat intake—another reason to choose salmon or tuna instead of steak or a burger.

Benefits of Healthy Fats

Choosing the right type of fats can make a difference for your health. In one recent study, for example, higher levels of EPA and DHA—the primary omega-3 fats found in fish and fish oil—were associated with a lower risk of death from all causes. Women with higher levels of EPA and DHA also had a lower risk of developing cardiovascular disease. Men with the highest levels of linoleic acid—an unsaturated fat that's the main component of soybean, canola, and corn oils—were 41 percent less likely to die of all causes than those with the lowest levels.

Another study found that higher blood levels of omega-3s from seafood as well as plant foods were associated with a lower risk of dying from heart attacks. People with the highest blood levels of omega-3s had about a 25 percent lower risk of fatal heart attack, compared to people with the lowest levels.

Consuming a small amount of healthy fats can even help you get more nutrients out of the vegetables you eat. In one study, starting at a bit less than a teaspoon of oil, increasing amounts of

Updated Nutrition Facts Panel

The new Nutrition Facts label drops "Calories from fat" and adds "Added sugars," recognizing recent research showing that not all fats are equally to be avoided and that added sugars should be limited.

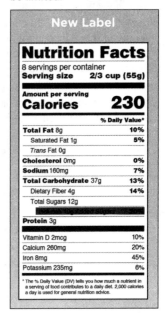

Sources of Saturated Fat

According to research conducted by the National Cancer Institute, these 10 foods contribute more than 50 percent of the saturated fat consumed in the U.S.:

- Regular cheese
- Pizza
- Grain-based desserts (pies, cakes)
- Dairy desserts (ice cream, cheesecake)
- Chicken and chicken mixed dishes
- Sausage, franks, bacon, and ribs
- Burgers
- Mexican mixed dishes
- Beef and beef mixed dishes

Not all of these foods are extremely high in saturated fat; rather, it's the quantity of these foods that Americans consume, combined with their saturated fat content, that puts them on the list. Note that many items on this list are prepared, processed foods.

Another way to look at it is to consider individual foods that are high in saturated fat, including some (like lamb) that are not consumed in significant quantities in the typical American diet. You'll see that some of these also appear on the previous list:

- Fatty cuts of beef (ribeye, T-bone, porterhouse, prime rib)
- Fatty cuts of pork (ribs, shoulder, butt, belly)
- Ground beef and pork that is less than 90% lean
- Processed meats (sausage, bacon, salami, hot dogs)
- Lamb
- Veal
- Poultry with skin
- Lard
- Cream
- Butter
- Whole milk and foods made from whole milk, including cheese (especially hard cheeses), yogurt, and ice cream
- Pizza
- Mexican and other mixed dishes, especially those including cheese and beef
- Grain- and dairy-based desserts

oil in test salads steadily boosted the levels of vitamins participants absorbed when they ate the salad. The maximum amount of oil used was about 7 teaspoons (a bit more than 2 tablespoons, containing 288 calories). The findings may help to explain why unsaturated oils support a healthy dietary pattern.

Fats and Diabetes Risk

An analysis of more than 100 randomized trials reported that swapping healthy unsaturated fats for carbohydrates or saturated fats also may reduce your risk of diabetes. Dariush Mozaffarian, MD, DrPH, dean of Tufts' Friedman School and senior author on the study, commented, "Our findings support preventing and treating insulin resistance and diabetes by eating more fat-rich foods like walnuts, sunflower seeds, soybeans, flaxseed, fish, and vegetable oils and spreads in place of refined grains, starches, sugars, and animal fats. This is a positive message for the public: Don't fear healthy fats."

The analysis found that eating more unsaturated fats, especially polyunsaturated fats, in place of either carbohydrates or saturated fats lowered blood sugar levels and improved insulin resistance and secretion. For every 5 percent of calories switched from carbohydrates or saturated fats to mono- or polyunsaturated fats, participants saw an approximately 0.1 unit improvement in HbA1c, a blood marker of long-term glucose control. Based on prior research, each 0.1 percent reduction in HbA1c is estimated to reduce the incidence of type 2 diabetes and cardiovascular diseases by 22 percent and 6.8 percent, respectively. Among different fats, the most consistent benefits were linked with increasing polyunsaturated fat intake.

Arthritis Associations

Switching from saturated to unsaturated fats also might be good for your aching joints. One study found that high intake of saturated fat was associated with a faster progression of knee osteoarthritis, while consuming more unsaturated fats was linked to slower progression. Study participants who reported the most saturated-fat intake were at 60 percent greater risk of osteoarthritis progression than those who consumed the least saturated fat. Those who reported the highest polyunsaturated fat consumption, on the other hand, were at 30 percent lower risk of osteoarthritis progression than those who consumed the least polyunsaturated fat.

"Following a healthy diet may be an effective strategy for knee osteoarthritis management, and is clearly more attractive than medications in terms of

Effects on Cholesterol

We've seen how scientists have revised their recommendations about dietary cholesterol and are debating the blood cholesterol effects of whole-fat dairy products. A similar debate has questioned the effects of saturated fat, leading to headlines like "Butter Is Back." As Tufts' Alice H. Lichtenstein, DSc, points out, however, "The conclusions of an extensive review—conducted by a group of researchers with an extensive range of backgrounds in the area of nutrition and cardiovascular disease risk, released by the American College of Cardiology and the American Heart Association—found strong evidence for a link between saturated fat (butter, cheese, fatty meat) and heart disease."

Saturated fats are found in animal products and tropical oils (palm, palm kernel, and coconut). It's clear that saturated fats composed of chains of 12 to 16 carbon atoms—including lauric acid, myristic acid, and palmitic acid—have the greatest effect on increasing LDL ("bad") cholesterol levels. In addition to raising LDL cholesterol, saturated fats also raise levels of HDL ("good") cholesterol, but not enough to offset the harmful effects of the higher LDL cholesterol. Sometimes, healthcare professionals speak of this in terms of the LDL/HDL cholesterol ratio: The lower the ratio—the more HDL cholesterol compared to LDL—the better.

So why the controversy? Part of the explanation may be what's consumed in place of saturated fat. Just as was seen with the "SnackWells effect," when fats are replaced by processed carbohydrates, the health benefits may be negated. So some experts caution that focusing on individual nutrients may never solve heart disease; saturated fat, for example, is only one contributor to heart disease. Your overall dietary pattern is more important than concerning yourself with single nutrients or foods.

"When considering different components of the diet, it is rarely an either/or situation," Dr. Lichtenstein notes. "When one component of the diet increases, another decreases. Choosing to focus on one, and not the other, can result in questionable conclusions."

Banning Trans Fat

On the other hand, there is no debate about the dangers of trans fats, now thought to be the worst type of fat for heart health. Trans fat is formed when hydrogen is added to liquid vegetable oils during food manufacturing, creating "partially hydrogenated oils" that remain solid at room temperature, which increase the food's shelf life and give it a more appealing texture. ("Fully" or "completely" hydrogenated oils do not contain trans fat.) Ironically, trans fat products were once hailed as a healthy alternative to butter and shortening. But now we know that trans fat increases LDL cholesterol and, unlike saturated fat, does not increase HDL cholesterol.

Experts advise avoiding manmade trans fat altogether. In 2018, the FDA largely banned trans fat from most food products, ruling such fats are no longer considered "generally recognized as safe."

Choosing Cooking Oil

The most direct way you might make decisions about the fat content of your diet comes when choosing cooking oils. Keep in mind that all popular oils contain a mix of different fatty acids. You might be tempted to buy only olive oil, which is high in monounsaturated fats, because of its role in the Mediterranean-style diet. But don't overlook liquid vegetable oils high in polyunsaturated fats, which may have their own health benefits.

Polyunsaturated Fats in Oils

Common cooking oils vary in their percentage of healthy polyunsaturated fat (primarily linoleic acid). Here are some popular choices ranked from most to least:

- Safflower oil 78%
- Sunflower oil 69%
- Corn oil 62%
- Soybean oil 61%
- Peanut oil 34%
- Canola oil 29%
- Lard 12%
- Palm oil 10%
- Olive oil 9%
- Butterfat 4%
- Palm kernel oil 2%
- Coconut oil 2%

Canola oil and olive oil are high in monounsaturated fat, which has been associated with health benefits in a Mediterranean-style diet. Lard, palm oil, butter, palm kernel oil, and coconut oil are high in saturated fat, which can raise your blood cholesterol levels.

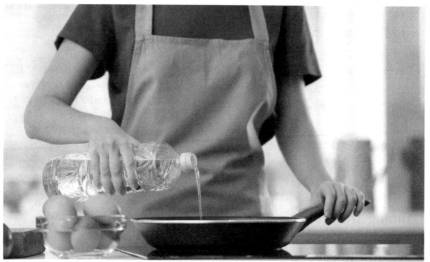

© Chernetskaya | Dreamstime

Use vegetable oil rather than butter when cooking.

Linoleic acid is the primary polyunsaturated fatty acid in the Western diet, found in liquid vegetable oils such as soybean, sunflower, safflower, and corn oils, as well as nuts and seeds. Research has found that people who swapped 5 percent of the calories they consumed from saturated fat sources such as red meat and butter with foods containing linoleic acid had a 9 percent lower risk of coronary heart disease events and a 13 percent lower mortality risk from coronary heart disease. Similar benefits were seen for swapping linoleic acid in place of calories from carbohydrates.

Other research suggests that omega-6 fats, such as linoleic acid, found in vegetable oils also may help reduce diabetes risk. In a long-term Finnish study, men with the highest blood levels of omega-6 fats were 60 percent less likely to develop type 2 diabetes than those with the lowest blood levels.

A tablespoon of soybean or corn oil contains about 7 to 8 grams of linoleic acid, and seven shelled walnuts provide about 11 grams. Consuming about two to three tablespoons of vegetable oil daily will provide you with enough linoleic acid to meet the Institute of Medicine's Adequate Intake recommendations of 14 grams per day for men over age 50 and 11 grams per day for women over age 50.

Dr. Lichtenstein cautions, "The emphasis should be on replacing animal fat with these sources of linoleic acid, not on adding sources of linoleic acid-rich foods or oils to the diet."

Fat Fads

Fats are almost as popular as protein and carbs when it comes to misinformation and half-truths online, in marketing hype, and in virtually every type of media. If scientists are still debating how different types of fat affect heart disease risk—the subject of countless large-scale studies—it's unlikely that these catchy but often baseless assertions are worthy of dietary changes. Here's a look at some popular notions as yet unproven by the evidence:

Claim: Monounsaturated fat is healthier than polyunsaturated because it doesn't oxidize.

"There is little evidence to support this claim," says Dr. Lichtenstein. "Most of the data suggest a stronger inverse association between polyunsaturated fatty acids and risk of cardiovascular disease than monounsaturated fatty acids."

Claim: Some fats fight inflammation and free radicals.

You may read about various fats, such as palmitic acid, having antioxidant or anti-inflammatory properties. Whatever (as yet unproven) benefits these antioxidants might have in fighting free radicals can't outweigh saturated fat's effects on increasing LDL cholesterol, however.

Claim: Saturated fat changes LDL cholesterol from small, dense, and very harmful molecules to large LDL molecules, which are benign.

Says Tufts' Dr. Lichtenstein, "The data on this are interesting but limited, and it is unclear how generalizable the available data are. There have been no intervention studies that show changing LDL particle size decreases heart disease risk—but there have been intervention studies that show replacing saturated fats with polyunsaturated fats decreases rates of cardiovascular disease."

Claim: Short- and medium-chain fats are metabolized differently than long-chain fats and contribute to improved satiety and increased fat burning.

"It is an interesting hypothesis; however, I have not seen adequate data to support the claim," says Dr. Lichtenstein. This claim is often made for lauric acid, a medium-chain fat found in coconut oil. (Short-chain fatty acids contain fewer than six carbons in length, while medium-chain fatty acids contain six to 12 carbons, and long-chain fatty acids have 14 to 24 carbons.) It's true that some small studies using pure, medium-chain fatty acids have shown a modest reduction in body weight, but studies actually using coconut oil (which is 44 percent lauric acid) have not achieved similar results.

Crazy for Coconut Oil

The most prevalent fat fad concerns coconut oil, which 72 percent of consumers consider as being healthy, according to one survey. Coconut oil is the subject of so many unsubstantiated claims that it merits a separate reality check.

The American Heart Association (AHA) has even sought to hit the brakes on the health claims for coconut oil. The association issued an advisory based on an analysis of more than 100 studies reaffirming that saturated fat raises unhealthy LDL cholesterol levels—specifically pointing out that coconut oil is mostly saturated fat. One tablespoon of coconut oil contains more than 11 grams of saturated fat—just shy of the AHA's recommended limit of 13 grams for an entire day.

It's true that a smattering of evidence suggests that the medium-chain triglycerides (MCTs) in coconut oil affect the body differently than the long-chain saturated fats generally found in animal fats. And some research hints that coconut oil may be helpful in reducing abdominal fat and blood sugar levels as well as increasing "good" HDL cholesterol levels. Experts advise, however, that the evidence is not strong enough to recommend using a lot of coconut oil in your diet.

In fact, the scientist behind much of the popular coconut oil claims echoed the AHA's cautionary advisory. That scientist's research used a special 100-percent MCT coconut oil, equivalent to consuming 10 tablespoons of coconut oil in a day. A subsequent study found coconut oil did not improve cardiometabolic risk factors or increase metabolism in overweight women.

As for brain-boosting claims for coconut oil, one study did report that coconut oil helped protect mouse cortical cells in the lab, but this finding does not translate to the conclusion that coconut oil is similarly good for human brains.

A Final Word on Fats

So what's the takeaway message on fats? Don't obsess about this fat or that one, and don't fret about limiting your total fat intake—as long as the total amount of calories from all sources doesn't exceed your needs. Eating more whole, plant-based foods and fewer animal-based foods and processed foods will ensure you're getting more unsaturated fats and fewer saturated and trans fats, without the need for counting fat grams.

The fat choices in your diet can affect your health, but you also need to give attention to reducing refined carbohydrates and added sugars. An overall dietary pattern that supports healthy aging is more important than whether you use an extra teaspoon of olive oil or choose soybean or corn oil at the supermarket. And no amount of coconut oil will cure cancer or guarantee that you'll live to be 100.

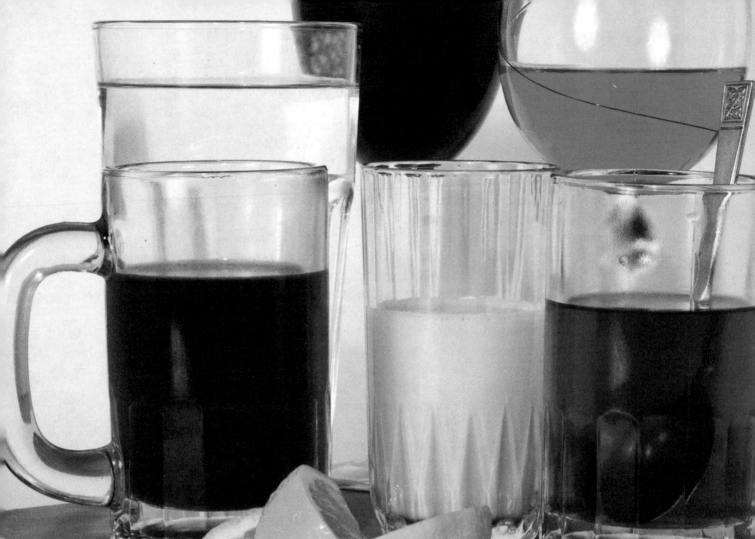

Water, coffee, tea, low-fat or fat-free milk, and wine (in moderation) are the healthiest beverage choices.

11 Better Beverages

You've no doubt heard about the supposed need to drink eight glasses of water a day and seen people toting plastic water bottles everywhere. In reality, you don't need to spend too much time monitoring your water intake or turning yourself into a camel. For most people, according to the Institute of Medicine, "fluid intake, driven by thirst… allows maintenance of hydration status and total body water at normal levels."

It is true, however, that you may be more likely to neglect your body's needs for water and other fluids as you get older. Older people often have a reduced sensation of thirst, so it's easier to miss the warning signs that you're becoming dehydrated.

Older individuals also tend to have lower reserves of fluid in their bodies, may eat less regularly, and may drink insufficient water following fluid deprivation to replenish their fluid deficit. Because of this, older people may need to pay more attention to their fluid intake, particularly during hot weather, and may need to drink fluids regularly, even if they are not thirsty.

Fluid Recommendations

The Adequate Intake (AI) of fluid is actually *more* than the popular notion of eight cups a day. But that's deceptive, because the AI includes water from all food and beverage sources—not just guzzling from water bottles. For men over age 50, the AI is 3.7 liters (almost 4 quarts) a day, which includes about 13 cups from beverages including water; the rest is typically obtained from food.

For women over age 50, the AI is 2.7 liters (a little less than 3 quarts) a day, with about 9 cups coming from water and other beverages.

Despite what you may have heard, the water in caffeinated beverages such as coffee and tea does count toward keeping you hydrated. So does the fluid content of foods, which can contribute significantly to your daily fluid intake.

Hydration Basics

To ensure that you're obtaining enough fluids, eat regular meals and drink plenty of water. And eat plenty of produce with a high water content—fruits like watermelon, grapes, melon, and oranges, and vegetables like cucumbers, celery, cauliflower, and lettuce.

Avoid sports drinks such as Gatorade unless you're engaged in extended vigorous activity in hot weather. Other sugar-sweetened beverages, such as sodas, sweetened tea and coffee drinks, and energy drinks aren't healthy choices.

In addition to drinking plenty of water and other healthy liquids to avoid dehydration, you can reduce your risk of becoming dehydrated by exercising regularly. Fit people of any age sweat more, keeping the body cool, but they also have more diluted sweat, losing fewer electrolytes as they perspire.

Dehydration Danger Signs

Especially as you get older, you may not recognize the warning signs of dehydration until you're in danger. Signs of dehydration include:

- Decreased urine output
- Dark-yellow or amber-colored urine
- Dry, sticky mouth
- Dry skin that doesn't spring back when pinched
- Sleepiness
- Headache
- Feeling dizzy or lightheaded
- Rapid heartbeat and/or breathing.

Why Nothing Beats Water

As we'll see, some plant-based beverages offer nutrients with health benefits, but your best daylong choice for staying hydrated is still plain water. It contains zero calories and has none of the potential downsides of drinking alcohol or sugary beverages. Best of all, water is virtually free—most municipal drinking water in the U.S. is safe, meaning you don't need to spend money on bottled or filtered water.

Water makes up most of your body, ranging from about 75 percent of body weight in infancy to 55 percent of body weight in older age. Your brain and heart are almost three-quarters water, your muscles and kidneys are almost 80 percent water, and even your bones are about 30 percent water. Every cell in your body needs water to function. Water transports nutrients and oxygen throughout your body and flushes away waste materials.

Your kidneys work more efficiently when your body has plenty of water; if they are deprived of adequate fluids, your kidneys must work harder. Recurrent dehydration can lead to kidney damage.

Your brain needs water to manufacture hormones and neurotransmitters. Research on the effects of dehydration on the brain is inconsistent, however, with short-term fluid deficiencies appearing to have the greatest impact on your mood and alertness.

Other ways in which your body uses water include:

- Serving as a "shock absorber" for your brain and spinal cord
- Lubricating your joints
- Making saliva for food consumption and digestion
- Keeping mucosal membranes moist; these include membranes in your mouth, nose, eyelids, windpipe, lungs, stomach, intestines, and urinary system.

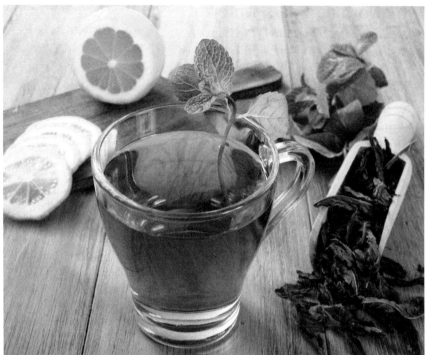
© Denio Rigacci | Dreamstime

In studies, drinking tea has been linked with several health benefits.

evidence that links good hydration with a reduced risk of kidney stones and other stones in the urinary system.

Benefits from Tea

Foods aren't the only way to get important nutrients as you age—certain beverages also can contribute beneficial nutrients while helping keep you hydrated. You can think of these beverages as a form of "liquid plants," since they are derived from plants and retain many of their sources' healthy nutrients, especially the phytonutrients. The most convincing evidence linking plant-based beverages to reduced risks of chronic diseases relates to tea and coffee. When you brew a cup of tea or a mug of coffee, you are extracting many of the nutrients from the tea leaves or coffee beans.

"If there's anything that can confidently be communicated to the public, it's the strong association of tea drinking with a lower risk of common chronic diseases, particularly heart disease, and the demonstration of that benefit through clinical trials," says Tufts expert Jeffrey Blumberg, PhD, who chaired an international symposium on tea and human health.

"About one-third of the weight of a tea leaf is flavonoids, which is high, especially when you consider that they are accompanied by virtually no calories," Dr. Blumberg explains. "There are a lot of related flavonoids in fruit and vegetables, but many people aren't consuming the amount of flavonoids in their diets as are being found necessary to promote health. Another way to get them is tea. A cup of tea is like adding a serving of fruit or vegetables to your diet."

It's possible to get too much of a good thing, especially if you're sensitive to caffeine. But tea contains about half the caffeine of coffee, and most of tea's benefits can be derived from decaffeinated teas (though some of the flavonoids are lost in the decaffeination process).

How Water Helps

Fluids including water can help prevent or ease constipation when coupled with increased fiber intake. In your intestines, fiber needs adequate fluid to create bulkier, softer stools and help keep stools moving. If you increase your fiber intake but don't get enough fluids, the fiber could cause constipation rather than easing it.

If you suffer from osteoarthritis, staying hydrated can help fight the inflammation associated with that disease. The Arthritis Foundation recommends "prehydrating"—drinking water before you exercise, not just after you've worked up a sweat—to help people with arthritis engage in physical activity with less discomfort. Increasing fluid intake also may help reduce the recurrence of gout.

On the other hand, ignore the claims of "water cures" touted in popular magazines, websites, and books: You can't "cure" heart disease, diabetes, cancer, or chronic pain simply by drinking lots of water. In fact, even the evidence linking healthy hydration to reduced risks of chronic diseases or conditions is relatively thin. The exception is strong

Research on Tea

Studies have found that tea drinking seems to benefit both your heart and brain. One study reported that drinking three cups of tea daily was associated with an 11 percent drop in the risk of heart attacks. Research on green tea has suggested that it might play a role in reducing the risks of stroke and death from cardiovascular disease and improving total and LDL cholesterol levels.

Studies also have linked tea drinking to beneficial effects on blood pressure. For example, men with high blood pressure who drank just one cup of black tea daily lowered their blood pressure, even when they ate a meal of foods that tend to constrict blood vessels and boost blood pressure.

Don't overlook herbal teas, which don't contain caffeine. Hibiscus, a common ingredient in herbal teas, is rich in antioxidants including anthocyanins, flavones, flavonols, and phenolic acids. Research led by Tufts' Diane L. McKay, PhD, scientific advisor for this Special Health Report, has shown that a few cups a day of herbal tea containing hibiscus can help lower high blood pressure as effectively as some medications do.

Lowering blood pressure might also have brain benefits, but that's not the only way tea seems to help protect your brain as you age. A phytonutrient in green tea, epigallocatechin-3-gallate, has antioxidant and anti-inflammatory properties that are believed to benefit brain function. Several animal studies have suggested that green tea extracts enhance learning and memory.

Evidence from human studies suggests a link between the nutrients in tea and improved memory, as well as a possible protective effect against Alzheimer's disease.

Good News on Coffee

If your mother warned that coffee was a health risk that could "stunt your growth," she'd be surprised to learn that coffee is now recognized as another "plant food" that can benefit your health. The 2015-2020 *Dietary Guidelines for Americans* mentions coffee specifically: Drinking three to five 8-ounce cups a day (up to about 400 milligrams of caffeine) is associated with minimal health risks and possible benefits, according to the experts.

Recently, two large studies reported that drinking coffee is associated with a modestly (less than 20 percent) reduced risk of dying from various conditions, compared to not drinking coffee.

In both studies, people who reported drinking coffee when they enrolled in the research were less likely than those who didn't drink coffee to have died during the follow-up period. Greater risk reduction generally was associated with daily intakes of two to three cups or more. The findings held regardless of ethnicity or where people lived and after adjusting for diet, lifestyle, and health status (like smoking and weight). In one study, coffee drinking was associated with a decreased risk of dying from heart disease, cancer, respiratory disease, stroke, diabetes, and kidney disease. In the other study, coffee drinkers had a decreased risk of dying from digestive diseases, including liver disease (men and women) and circulatory diseases, like heart disease and stroke (particularly women).

Coffee vs. Diabetes

Other research has linked increasing coffee consumption with lower risk of developing diabetes. Participants who increased their coffee intake by more than one 8-ounce cup per day over a four-year period were 11 percent less likely to be diagnosed with diabetes during the subsequent four years. On the other hand, people who decreased their coffee consumption by more than a cup per day were at 17 percent greater risk of type 2 diabetes.

NEW FINDING

Coffee Drinkers May Live Longer

Further evidence for the health benefits of coffee consumption comes from a large Spanish study involving 19,888 participants and a total of more than 200,000 person-years of follow-up. During the span of the study, 337 participants died from all causes. Overall, consuming an additional two cups of coffee per day was associated with a 22 percent lower mortality risk. The connection was strongest for participants ages 55 and older. Another study of about a half-million Britons reported similar findings, while also countering previous research linking coffee benefits to the speed at which a person metabolizes caffeine. During a 10-year follow-up period, some 14,200 participants died. Coffee consumption was associated with reduced mortality risk, including those drinking filtered, instant, and decaffeinated coffee, and regardless of the rate of caffeine metabolism. Compared to non-coffee drinkers, those who drank one cup daily saw an eight percent reduced risk of mortality, which improved to 16 percent for those drinking six to seven cups.

American Journal of Clinical Nutrition, November 2018
JAMA Internal Medicine, August 2018

Researchers credited phytonutrients in coffee with the apparent benefit—not the caffeine. They noted that effects on glucose metabolism have previously been found in studies of decaffeinated coffee.

Calming A-fib Fears

What about worries that the caffeine in coffee might increase the risk of atrial fibrillation (A-fib, a type of abnormal heart rhythm that can increase the risk of stroke)? Coffee is best known for its stimulating effect that boosts alertness, improves focus, and increases productivity. For some people, however, too much coffee causes "jitters," and some health experts have voiced concerns that too much stimulation might contribute to A-fib. Researchers who studied this possibility found little reason for worry, however: A meta-analysis concluded that it's unlikely habitual caffeine intake from coffee and other dietary sources increases A-fib risk. In fact, the analysis found that A-fib risk fell with increasing caffeine intake.

Pros and Cons of Alcohol

The health picture is more complicated for another popular type of beverage—alcohol, such as wine, beer, and spirits. On the plus side, moderate alcohol consumption has been linked to a reduced risk of cardiovascular disease, and the resveratrol compounds in red wine are being studied for a wide range of health effects. Moderate drinking also may reduce osteoporosis risk in postmenopausal women by slowing the rate of bone "remodeling"—the body's ongoing replacement of old bone with new.

According to a study in *Diabetologia*, frequent—but not heavy—alcohol consumption might reduce the risk of developing diabetes. The large study followed more than 70,000 Danish men and women for almost five years. Compared to non-drinkers, women who consumed nine alcoholic beverages a week had a 58 percent lower diabetes risk, and men who consumed 14 drinks a week had a 43 percent lower risk than teetotalers. The findings aren't a license to overdo alcohol, however: Researchers reported a U-shaped curve in associations between drinking and diabetes risk, with the lowest risk in the middle (moderate, frequent consumption) and higher risk both for non-drinkers and heavy drinkers. Men and women who drank alcohol three to four days a week were at lowest risk.

When making decisions about alcohol consumption, don't overlook the array of harmful effects that may result from alcohol abuse and dependence. The 2015-2020 *Dietary Guidelines for Americans* advises women who choose to drink alcoholic beverages to limit intake to one glass a day and men to limit their intake to two drinks. Excessive alcohol consumption has health consequences including liver damage and increased cancer risk, as well as social, psychological, and legal risks.

Alcohol and Aging

Even if you could "hold your liquor" when you were younger, your body's ability to metabolize alcohol declines with age; this is especially true with women. This means that older adults need to be especially cautious with their alcohol use. According to AARP, one in 10 older adults who drink alcohol are at risk of excessive or potentially harmful alcohol use. In older adults, alcohol also is more likely to interact with medications, which may interfere with or amplify the drugs' intended effects.

The National Institute on Alcohol Abuse and Alcoholism (NIAAA) suggests that people over age 65 limit themselves to no more than one alcoholic drink a day, and not more than two on any occasion. High levels of alcohol in the body can mask or worsen symptoms of stroke, diabetes, memory loss, heart disease, or mood disorders.

Alcoholic beverages also provide a significant number of calories without contributing any important nutrients. A 12-ounce glass of beer has about 150 calories, a 5-ounce glass of red wine has about 125 calories, and a 1.5-ounce shot of liquor has about 100 calories, according to the NIAAA. Your brain doesn't process the signals from beverage calories the same way it does from food calories, so drinking doesn't decrease feelings of hunger. Instead, it can loosen your inhibitions and lead to excess eating or snacking.

Skip Sugary Beverages

Sugary beverages such as soft drinks account for almost half the added sugar in the American diet. These beverages also include sports drinks, energy drinks, "gourmet" tea and coffee drinks, and juice drinks that are not 100-percent fruit juice. Such beverages are major contributors to the obesity epidemic. It doesn't matter what sweetener is used: High-fructose corn syrup, dextrose, honey, evaporated cane juice, agave nectar, and many other forms of sugar all contain calories and affect the body similarly.

Sugary beverages can quickly add up to meet or exceed the dietary guidelines' limit on added sugars of less than 10 percent of calories per day. In a 2,000-calorie daily diet, that means no more than 200 calories from added sugars, or roughly 12 teaspoons—about the amount in just one regular 16-ounce soft drink.

Health Effects

The risks of consuming sugar-sweetened drinks are not limited to putting on a few pounds. These beverages also contribute to conditions linked with obesity, including cardiovascular disease and type 2 diabetes. For example, people who averaged seven non-diet soda servings per week—just one a day—were 29 percent more likely to die from cardiovascular causes than those consuming less.

Tufts researchers have reported that sugary drinks may also increase your odds of developing non-alcoholic fatty liver disease (NAFLD). NAFLD, which is characterized by a buildup of fat in the liver unrelated to alcohol consumption, may cause the liver to swell and become inflamed, which can lead to scarring (cirrhosis) and, eventually, to liver failure. CT scans showed a higher prevalence of NAFLD among people who reported drinking more than one sugar-sweetened beverage per day compared to people who said they drank none.

Debating Diet Soda

You may be tempted to avoid sugary beverages simply by choosing a "diet" version of the same type of drink. However, concerns also have been raised about the safety of non-caloric sweeteners such as aspartame used in diet sodas. Some have suggested that

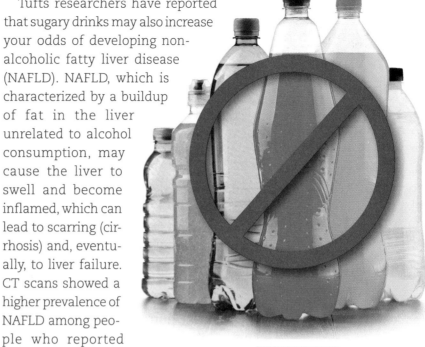

© Paulcocken | Dreamstime

Sugar-sweetened beverages include many bottled juice drinks, energy drinks, and tea drinks, as well as soft drinks.

Sugary Drinks Raise Risks

The more sugar-sweetened beverages people drink, the greater their risk of premature death, according to a large, long-term study of U.S. adults. The risk of early death linked with drinking sugary beverages was more pronounced among women. The Harvard study also found that drinking one artificially sweetened "diet" beverage per day instead of a sugary one was linked with a lower risk of premature death. However, drinking four or more diet drinks per day was associated with an increased risk of mortality in women. Researchers analyzed data from 80,647 women participating in the Nurses' Health Study (1980-2014) and 37,716 men in the Health Professionals Follow-Up Study (1986-2014). For both studies, participants answered questionnaires about their lifestyles and health status every two years. The more sugary drinks a person drank, the more the risk of early death from any cause increased. Compared with drinking sugary drinks less than once per month, drinking one to two per day was associated with a 14 percent increase in risk, and two or more per day with a 21 percent increase in risk.

Circulation, April 30, 2019

non-caloric sweeteners might somehow contribute to weight gain. One study even linked diet soda consumption to increased stroke and dementia risk.

According to the FDA, however, "Food safety experts generally agree there is no convincing evidence of a cause-and-effect relationship between these sweeteners and negative health effects in humans." While it's best not to overdo diet drinks, based on current evidence, artificial sweeteners remain an acceptable option for people who are working to control their weight—but water or unsweetened coffee, tea, or low-fat milk are healthier choices.

Cola Caution

Cola drinks, whether sugared or diet, may present special concerns about bone health, especially for postmenopausal women. In one study, women who drank three or more cola drinks daily had lower bone mineral density (BMD) in areas of bones that are common sites for fractures. In men, however, there was no link between cola consumption and lower BMDs, and consumers of non-cola soft drinks did not have lower BMDs.

Phosphoric acid, an ingredient found in cola drinks but not other flavors of sodas, might be to blame. In addition, caffeine, also found in colas but not most other soft drinks, can interfere with calcium absorption, and the study found a greater decrease in bone density among caffeinated soda drinkers.

Another factor may simply be that people who drink soft drinks and sweetened beverages of any type tend to drink less milk, which reduces their intake of calcium necessary to build healthy bones. If you're an all-day soda drinker, consider substituting water for some of those sodas.

Eating for Healthy Aging

Making smart choices—whether beverages or foods—as part of an overall healthy dietary pattern is increasingly important as you get older. Following a scientifically proven nutrition plan such as that shown in Tufts' MyPlate for Older Adults can help you lower your risks of illness and live healthier longer.

While minimizing your risks of chronic diseases is a lifelong concern, as you get older, this concern inevitably looms larger. As peers, friends, and loved ones are diagnosed with chronic conditions more common among older adults, it's natural to wonder: What can I do to improve my odds? As we've seen throughout this book, with many of these conditions, making healthy modifications to your diet can protect you as you age.

It's never too late to benefit from eating better, and there's no better time to start than right now.

alpha-linolenic acid (ALA): An essential fatty acid that, along with EPA and DHA, belongs to a group of fats called omega-3 fatty acids. EPA and DHA are found primarily in fish, while ALA is found in plant seeds and oils such as flaxseed, canola, soy and walnut oils. ALA is also found in walnuts and in wild plants like purslane. The body converts some ALA to EPA and DHA, which are more easily used by the body.

anthocyanins: A type of flavonoid in plants that acts as a pigment, giving many common fruits and vegetables their color.

antioxidants: A substance in the blood that protect cells from damage caused by harmful unstable molecules produced in response to stress or exposure to environmental toxins. Antioxidants include flavonoids, beta-carotene, lycopene, selenium, and vitamins A, C, and E. Many more compounds in fruits, vegetables, legumes, nuts, and whole grains are antioxidants.

body mass index (BMI): A calculation that combines weight and height: (Weight in Pounds / [Height in inches x Height in inches]) x 703. A BMI of over 25 is considered overweight, and over 30 is obese.

carbohydrates: Compounds of carbon, hydrogen, and oxygen that form sugars, starches, and cellulose; carbohydrates are one of the body's main sources of energy.

cholesterol: A waxy, fat-like substance found in foods of animal origin and synthesized by the body that can contribute to artherosclerosis ("hardening of the arteries"), but that is secondary to saturated fat. In the blood, serum cholesterol combines with proteins to form LDL and HDL cholesterol. Serum cholesterol can contribute to plaque buildup in the arteries.

DASH diet: The Dietary Approaches to Stop Hypertension eating plan is high in fruits, vegetables, and grains, while low in meat, sweets, and salt. This diet was designed and tested in a clinical tudy that examined the effects of a specific way of eating on blood pressure. Study results suggest that you can lower high blood pressure with an eating plan that emphasizes fruits, vegetables, low-fat dairy foods, whole grains, poultry, fish, and nuts. The diet is low in saturated fat, total fat, and cholesterol.

docosahexaenoic acid (DHA): A type of omega-3 fatty acid found in fish and algae that is essential for heart and brain health. (See also: omega-3 fatty acid.)

eicosapentaenoic acid (EPA): A type of omega-3 fatty acid found in fish that is essential for heart and brain health. (See also: omega-3 fatty acid.)

fats: Compounds containing fatty acids, which may be monounsaturated, polyunsaturated, or saturated.

flavonoids: A group of more than 5,000 antioxidant compounds naturally present in vegetables, fruits, and beverages like tea, red wine, and fruit juices, and known for a dazzling array of pigments. Research suggests flavonoids may protect against damage to blood vessels, decreasing the risk of cardiovascular disease. In addition, they may have a role in cancer prevention and help boost the immune system.

glucose: A sugar used by the body as a source of energy. Food that is eaten is broken down in the digestive system into glucose.

high-density lipoprotein (HDL) cholesterol: Often referred to as "good" cholesterol, HDL cholesterol reduces cholesterol buildup in the arteries, thereby reducing the risk of heart disease. (See also: cholesterol, Low-density lipoprotein [LDL] cholesterol.)

insulin: A hormone released by the pancreas that causes cells to take up sugar (glucose) from the bloodstream to use and store for energy. Insulin is important in carbohydrate, fat, and protein metabolism.

insulin resistance: Reduced sensitivity to insulin that is typical of type 2 diabetes, but also may occur in the absence of diabetes.

lipids: Fats or fat-like substances. Lipid levels in the bloodstream are commonly measured to evaluate cardiovascular health risks. Lipids include LDL cholesterol, HDL cholesterol, and triglycerides.

lipoprotein: A specialized, microscopic, spherical particle in the blood composed of protein and lipids. Its role is to move lipids from one part of the body to another.

low-density lipoprotein (LDL) cholesterol: Often referred to as "bad" cholesterol, LDL cholesterol transports cholesterol to the arteries, where it can build up and lead to heart disease. They contain more fat and less protein than HDL. They stick to artery walls and contribute to plaque buildup and, as a result, are linked to clogged arteries and coronary artery disease.

lycopene: The natural red pigment that gives tomatoes their color. Research suggests it is a powerful antioxidant that may have health benefits. Most of the lycopene in the diet comes from tomatoes, especially cooked tomato products such as canned tomatoes, spaghetti sauce and ketchup.

Mediterranean-style diet: A dietary style influenced by the traditional dietary patterns of Mediterranean countries, particularly Italy, Greece and Spain. It emphasizes olive oil as the primary source of dietary fat, an abundance of plant foods, including fruits and vegetables, whole grains, beans, nuts, and seeds, moderate amounts of fish and poultry each week and moderate amounts of cheese and yogurt each day. It traditionally includes a moderate amount of wine (one to two glasses per day for men, one for women).

monounsaturated fat: A type of healthy fat in which only one carbon atom is not bound to hydrogen (this is also called a "double bond"); monounsaturated fats, found in olive, walnut, canola, and other vegetable oils, are generally liquid at room temperature.

omega-3 fatty acids: Essential fatty acids found in fish, walnuts, soy products, and some seeds and vegetable oils that can reduce the risk of cardiovascular disease and may help protect brain function.

omega-6 fatty acids: A type of unsaturated fat found in many nuts, seeds, and vegetable oils, and in some poultry, seafood, and vegetables. One omega-6 fatty acid, linoleic acid, is essential to the body and is absorbed from our diet.

phytonutrients (also called phytochemicals): Compounds in plants that provide flavor, aroma, and color, and protect the plant from microbes and environmental damage. When consumed by humans, phytonutrients are believed to promote health and prevent disease.

polyphenols: A group of naturally occurring plant compounds, including flavonoids and isoflavones, with antioxidant properties that may benefit health.

polyunsaturated fat: A type of fat in which more than one carbon atom is not bound to hydrogen; polyunsaturated fats are healthy and generally liquid at room temperature, as in vegetable oil.

protein: Essential constituents of living cells; plant or animal tissue rich in such compounds, considered as a food source supplying essential amino acids to the body.

saturated fat: A type of fat that can increase unhealthy cholesterol levels and raise the risk of heart disease. Saturated fatty acids are found primarily in animal foods, especially meats and full-fat dairy products.

trans fat: A type of fat in processed foods that is manufactured by adding hydrogen to liquid oil to solidify it, resulting in the formation of a partially hydrogenated oil. Trans fat increases unhealthy LDL cholesterol levels and lowers healthy HDL cholesterol levels. Note: Trans fats were banned by the U.S. Food & Drug Administration in 2018.

whole grains: Grains that contain all the essential parts and naturally occurring nutrients of the entire grain seed—the bran, germ, and endosperm.

Academy of Nutrition and Dietetics
eatright.org
800-877-1600
120 S. Riverside Plaza, Suite 2190
Chicago, IL 60606-6995

American Cancer Society (ACS)
www.cancer.org
800-227-2345
50 Williams St. NW
Atlanta, GA 30303

American Diabetes Association (ADA)
diabetes.org
800-342-2383
2451 Crystal Dr., Suite 900
Arlington, VA 22202

American Heart Association
www.heart.org
800-242-8721
7272 Greenville Ave.
Dallas, TX 75231

American Institute for Cancer Research
aicr.org
800-843-8114
1560 Wilson Blvd., Suite 1000
Arlington, VA 22209

Dietary Guidelines for Americans 2015-2020
health.gov/dietaryguidelines/2015/guidelines/
240-453-8280

Office of Disease Prevention and Health Promotion
U.S. Department of Health and Human Services
1101 Wootton Pkwy., Suite LL100
Rockville, MD 20852

Environmental Working Group
www.ewg.org
202-667-6982
1436 U St. NW, Suite 100
Washington, DC 200099

Food and Diet Advice
www.choosemyplate.gov
This website by the U.S. Department of Agriculture
explains the *Dietary Guidelines for Americans*
and gives interactive assistance in helping
you decide what and how much to eat.

Food and Drug Administration
www.fda.gov
888-463-6332
10903 New Hampshire Ave.
Silver Spring, MD 20993

**Friedman School of Nutrition Science and Policy—
Tufts University**
nutrition.tufts.edu
617-636-3737
150 Harrison Ave.
Boston, MA 02111

**Jean Mayer USDA Human Nutrition
Research Center of Aging**
hnrca.tufts.edu
617-556-3000
711 Washington St.
Boston, MA 02111

National Cancer Institute (NCI)
www.cancer.gov
800-422-6237
BG 9609 MSC 9760
9609 Medical Center Dr.
Bethesda, MD 20892-9760

National Heart, Lung and Blood Institute (NHLBI)
www.nhlbi.nih.gov
Bldg 31
3131 Center Dr.
Bethesda, MD 20892

National Institutes of Health
nih.gov
301-496-4000
9000 Rockville Pike
Bethesda, MD 20892

National Institute on Aging
www.nia.nih.gov
(800) 222-2225; (800) 222-4225 (TTY)
Bldg 31, Rm 5C27
31 Center Dr., MSC 2292
Bethesda, MD 20892

Oldways Whole Grains Council
wholegrainscouncil.org
617-421-5500
266 Beacon St.
Boston, MA 02116

Tufts University *Health & Nutrition Letter*
www.nutritionletter.tufts.edu
PO Box 5656
Norwalk, CT 06856

Tufts' MyPlate for Older Adults
hnrca.tufts.edu/myplate

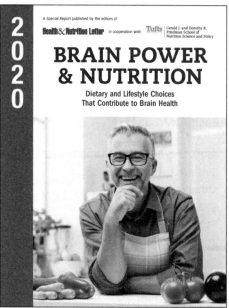
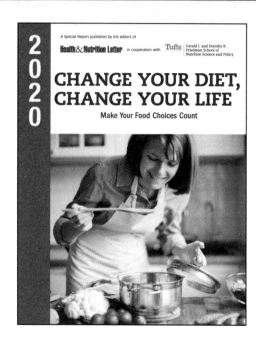
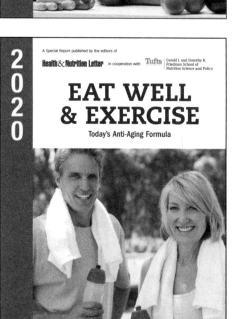
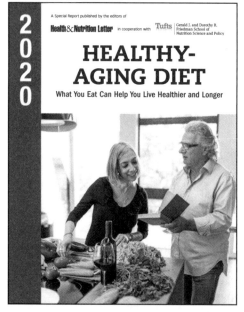
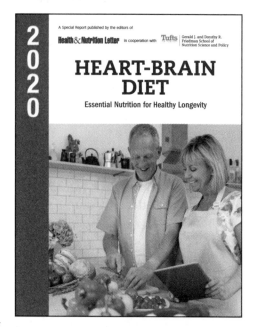
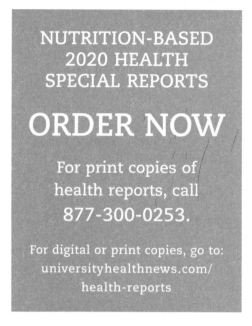